HarperCollins books may be purchased for educational, business, or sales promotional use. For information, please write: Special Markets Department, HarperCollins Publishers, Inc., 10 East 53rd Street, New York, NY 10022.

FIRST EDITION

Designed by Irving Perkins Associates
The illustrations and charts in this book were created using the following software: CorelDRAW 4.0, VISIO2.0, Lotus Freelance for Windows 2.0, and Eat Smart, Think Smart for Windows 1.0.

Library of Congress Cataloging-in-Publication Data
Haas, Robert, 1948–
    Eat smart, think smart: how to use nutrients and supplements to achieve maximum mental and physical performance/Robert Haas.—1st ed.
        p.   cm.
    Includes bibliographical references and index.
    ISBN 0-06-017044-1 (cloth)
    1. Nutrition.   2. Mental   efficiency—Nutritional   aspects.   3. Mental   work—Nutritional aspects.   I. Title.
    RA776.5.H224   1993
    613.2—dc20   93-37677

94   95   96   97   98   PS/RRD   10   9   8   7   6   5   4   3   2   1

*This book is dedicated to my parents,
who made me eat my smart nutrients every day*

Contents

Acknowledgments

I gratefully acknowledge the following people (in alphabetical order) for the time, effort, and expertise they offered during the research and writing of this book:

- Charlotte Abbott, for her excellent and thorough editorial comments and suggestions
- Wendy Almeleh, for a wonderful copyediting job
- Larry Ashmead, for his stewardship, editorial suggestions, and recognition of the importance of this book
- Steve Blechman (Twin Laboratories), for supplying data, nutrients, and continued support
- Connie Clausen, my literary mentor, who kept me focused through it all
- Steve Diamond, for his incomparable computer programming skills
- Michael Hoffman (Heart Communications), for product research information
- Guy Kettelhack, for his expert editorial assistance and organizational skills
- Life Fitness (LifeCycle) corporation, for helping to keep me fit during the writing of this book
- Kristin Massey, for her invaluable assistance, suggestions, and sustenance during the research, writing, and editing of this book
- Durk Pearson and Sandy Shaw, for their insightful thoughts, comments, and suggestions
- Hilarie Porter, for the delicious smart recipes and for being perfect, as usual
- Rosalyn and Chester Salamon, for their legal and literary assistance

Introduction

It's difficult to be a nutritional pioneer.

When my first book, *Eat to Win,* became the number 1 bestselling "how-to" book of the year in 1984 (according to the *New York Times* bestseller list and *Publishers Weekly*), a large constituency of scientists and physicians (not to mention book reviewers), who vehemently disagreed with and criticized my work, wound up looking foolish and embarrassingly unscientific. My critics and detractors couldn't accept the fact that they had so flagrantly misjudged the preponderance of published expert evidence. Yet my research and sports nutrition program, substantiated and validated by thousands of published journal articles over the past ten years, is *still* the nutritional gold standard for athletes the world over.

I expect that the book you now hold in your hands will create a similar scenario of rage, frenzy, and excitement: rage on the part of scientists—those who are unable to see beyond the limited horizon of their own ignorance or those who are unwilling to accept new ideas; frenzy on the part of ultra-conservative health organizations (desiring to maintain the nutritional status quo and their own political agendas) to get "friends" in the press to pan this book; excitement on the part of many intelligent lay readers, scientists, and physicians who understand the scientific truths and rationale behind the Eat Smart, Think Smart nutrition plans. It is for them that I wrote this book.

The Pursuit of Personal Excellence

This is, first and foremost, a book about *excellence.* It is for people from all walks of life—students, professors, Wall Street traders, air traffic controllers, research scientists, CEOs, managers, secretaries, artists, writers, entertainers, news commentators, crossword puzzlers, musicians, editors, and, of course, Generation X (those people aged 18–25 who have already embraced smart drinks and smart nutrients)—everyone who strives for mental fitness. If personal excellence through maximum mental performance is your goal, you've just made a wise investment by purchasing this book.

The Book for Your Brain

Weighing in at a mere three pounds—about 2 percent of your body's total weight—your brain devours 20 percent of your body's total energy supply and 20 percent of all the oxygen you inhale. Your brain has an insatiable and lifelong appetite for vitamins, minerals, amino acids, sugar (glucose), and oxygen.

Sadly, the vast majority of people who aspire to excellence probably don't feed their brains the right stuff. Many mistakenly believe that intelligence, memory, and overall mental performance are dictated by genetics, so why even try to boost their brain power?

Recent research has proved the opposite: Mind and mental processes are dynamic and fluid, changeable and improvable. Although the number of neurons (nerve cells) in the brain are fixed at birth (or shortly thereafter), the potential for improvement appears to be boundless. This book opens up the possibilities of mental growth, improvement, and brain antiaging through the use of smart nutrients from foods and nutritional supplements.

Why You Must Eat Smart to Think Smart

Your brain's nerve cells *never* reproduce. The cells lining your intestinal tract reproduce new offspring every two to three days, red blood cells are replaced every three to four months, and even bone cells reproduce within two to five years. Yet the brain does not renew its neurons. Does this fixed number of neurons place us at risk as we age?

Over time, your brain's neurons accumulate damage and cellular waste material caused chiefly by destructive atoms and molecules called free radicals. These molecular piranha destroy cell walls and DNA, causing all the consequences of premature brain aging—cell malfunction, memory loss, personality changes, senility, stroke, and cancer.

It is imperative, therefore, that you learn how to nourish and safeguard your fixed number of brain neurons because, quite simply, they are the only ones you've got and will ever have. You must learn how to eat smart not only to think smart, but to stay smart, healthy, and rational.

Approximately 15 percent of the oxygen we breathe combines with fats and other substances in the brain to form destructive free radicals. Fortunately, we have at our disposal an arsenal of antioxidant smart nutrients—B-complex vitamins, vitamins C, E, and beta-carotene; the minerals zinc and selenium; amino acids, such as L-cysteine; and the three-amino acid antioxidant molecule, L-glutathione. These smart nutrients have the power to neutralize free radicals, thereby preventing neuronal damage that leads to premature aging and diminished mental function. Many scientists now believe that each day of our lives, free radicals cause the primary damage that leads to memory loss, senility, and brain cancer. There's no time like the present to learn how to eat smart. This book will show you precisely how to do just that.

Why Haven't You Heard about Smart Nutrients Before?

Until the pioneering work of scientists at the Massachusetts Institute of Technology (MIT) in the 1970s and 80s, it was assumed that the levels of neurotransmitters in the brain (the chemicals used by the brain to control all cognitive functions) were controlled entirely by the brain. No one knew that vitamins, amino acids (the molecular building blocks of all proteins), and other nutrients could enhance cognitive functions. The MIT researchers were the first to demonstrate that levels of neurotransmitters in the brain could be significantly influenced by the nutrient composition of a *single meal.* They discovered, for example, that

1. A protein-rich meal can raise levels of the brain neurotransmitter norepinephrine, promoting increased alertness, assertiveness, and the ability to make decisions under pressure.
2. A meal rich in carbohydrates and low in protein can increase brain levels of the neurotransmitter serotonin, inducing a relaxed or even sleepy state.
3. The nutrient choline (found in seafood, legumes, and lecithin, for example), can raise brain acetylcholine levels, improving students' scores on memory tests.

Scientists have recently discovered that other nutrients and nutritional supplements help the brain manufacture its own smart drugs. The popular press has recently found a growing smart-nutrient underground movement in the United States. Known as Generation X, these smart-nutrient advocates substitute "smart drinks" for alcoholic beverages in smart bars from coast to coast. Television shows, such as "Nightline," "Larry King Live," "20/20," "Donahue," "Today," "Good Morning America," and publications, such as *USA Today, Time, Newsweek, Omni, Mondo 2000, Longevity,* and *Psychology Today,* have recently examined the beginnings of what I call the *smart nutrition revolution.*

Why Smart Nutrients?

No prescribed mind (psychotropic) drug in widespread use in the United States addresses the cause of deficiencies in neurotransmitters. Most drugs only stimulate a temporary release of preexisting stores of neurotransmitters; they do nothing to increase the production of neurotransmitters. This fact reveals why many drugs lose their effectiveness with chronic use: Once preexisting supplies of neurotransmitters are exhausted, these drugs are unable to stimulate the production and release of additional neurotransmitters.

Smart nutrients attack the problem of neurotransmitter deficiencies at its root. They supply the brain with the essential amino acids, vitamins, minerals, and nutrient cofactors that it needs to manufacture adequate amounts of neurotransmitter. If the smart-nutrient intake of all Americans was optimal, the widespread use of psychotropic drugs that are designed to treat depression, anxiety, senility, and personality disorders would greatly diminish—an enviable goal, given the side effects and addictive properties of these drugs, especially when combined with alcohol.

Smart drugs (technically called nootropics), used widely throughout Europe for years, have recently become popular in the United States. These drugs have not been approved by the Food and Drug Administration (FDA) and, accordingly, are not sold or prescribed in this country.

As you will discover, there is no clearly established evidence that apparently healthy, normal people need to take smart drugs (for completeness, I've discussed some of them in Chapter 8 and included manufacturers' addresses and phone numbers in Appendix I). Many of these drugs aren't necessary because many of them are based on the molecular formulas of the smart nutrients you'll learn about in this book—nutrients that you can find in foods and nutritional supplements for a fraction of the cost. Finally, nutrients, as a rule, appear to be safer alternatives to drugs (although the incidence of side effects from smart drugs is low, compared to those of many other prescription medications).

Of course, nothing is 100 percent safe: *everything, including air and water, is dangerous* in excessive amounts; for that reason, I strongly recommend that you consult with a physician before you begin any dietary plan, including those in this book. Your physician is the best judge of whether you should embrace any nutrition plan, and I urge you to be medically monitored until your physician is satisfied that you can safely follow your new dietary plan.

What Does the FDA Think about Smart Nutrients?

The FDA was created in 1938 (under the New Deal, a legislative plan devised at a time when more governmental regulation was thought to be desirable). Until that time, American citizens made their own health-care choices and were allowed to purchase whatever nutrients and drugs they desired. The drug laws of the time were designed to prevent fraud, not access. As surprising as it may sound today, in those days Americans purchased only about 5 percent of their drugs through prescriptions; the vast majority purchased all legal drugs over the counter. Within six months of its creation, the FDA removed many drugs from the over-the-counter market, making them available only by prescription.

Recently, nutritional supplements have come under FDA scrutiny to the point where the FDA has threatened to remove many of them, including smart nutrients, from the over-the-counter market. Amino acids, herbs, nonvitamin nutrients (such as coenzyme Q_{10}), and vitamin and mineral supplements that are well above the RDA (recommended dietary allowance) levels are on the FDA's acknowledged hit list. Why?

One scientist who served on an FDA advisory panel publicly admitted that, in general, the FDA harbors a bias against most, if not all, nutritional supplements. It should come as no surprise, then, that the FDA considers almost any scientifically valid health claims for nutritional supplements to be "mislabeling" and, therefore, a reason to remove them from the consumer market.

Until the 1980s, the FDA successfully stopped the general public from learning about the health benefits of specific nutrients in foods and dietary supplements by preventing manufacturers from making *any* health claims for the products. The advent of the personal computer; on-line information services, such as CompuServe, Prodigy, and the Internet; and the growing popularity of health-oriented publications, such as *Omni, Longevity,* and *American Health,* have made it possible for ordinary Americans to learn about the life-extending and mind-expanding properties of nutrients and nutritional supplements (see Appendixes II and IV to learn how you can use your personal computer to eat smart.

This situation, however, has evidently not changed the information-smothering policies of the FDA, which, for example, will not permit health claims for folic acid, a B vitamin that has been shown to prevent neural tube birth defects, including spina bifida. Research has shown that the incidence of infants born with neural tube defects is much lower among women who take folic acid supplements around the time of conception than among women who are deficient in folic acid. Ironically, the U.S. Public Health Service (the parent organization of the FDA) recommends that all women of childbearing age take folic acid supplements! Even though Congress passed the Nutrition and Education Labeling Act, which requires the FDA to consider permitting vitamin manufacturers to make the specific health claim for folic acid supplements regarding neural tube defects, the FDA did nothing, essentially ignoring the congressional mandate. The FDA has consistently refused to allow health claims for nutrients, including the ability of vitamin E and beta-carotene to prevent heart attacks and the association of dietary fiber intake with the decreased risk of colon cancer.

The FDA acts only to restrict information, not to provide it to help consumers make informed, intelligent decisions about drugs and nutrients. The FDA would like to remove most smart nutrients from the consumer market by reclassifying them as drugs. Once the pharmaceutical companies obtain a monopoly on the sale of nutritional supplements, you can expect the prices to soar.

Even if the FDA is successful in reclassifying some dietary supplements as drugs, this book will show you how to obtain all essential smart nutrients from ordinary foods, food combinations, and nutritional supplements. I've also provided a list of manufacturers and suppliers abroad who will, in all likelihood, sell smart nutrients to U.S. citizens should the FDA succeed in removing them from the consumer market (the FDA permits individuals to import a three-month personal supply of unapproved substances that are legal in their country of origin; see Appendix I for a list of manufacturers and their addresses and telephone numbers). I've even included an FDA Survival Guide (Appendix V) to show you how to obtain smart nutrients (or provide your body with the raw materials it can use to synthesize smart nutrients) from foods and available supplements if the FDA is successful in removing certain smart nutrients from the consumer market.

In all fairness, the FDA is in a tough position. It is the first entity blamed when an approved drug, such as thalidomide, causes harmful disfiguring and disabling birth defects. As the primary agency responsible for preventing fraudulent health claims for all drugs, food products, and dietary supplements, it must be ever vigilant to protect consumers from irresponsible and unscientific claims made by unscrupulous manufacturers for their products. The main problem is that the FDA harbors a general bias against nutritional supplements—even those that most credible scientists already know prevent bodily damage that can lead to degenerative diseases, such as heart attack, stroke, and certain types of cancer. Since the FDA will not allow food, drug, and supplement manufacturers to share this information with the general public, it's up to books, such as this one, to educate the lay consumer.

What the FDA Should Do

The dietary-supplement industry has its share of unethical individuals—but so does the pharmaceutical industry, the medical industry, the food industry, and just about every other health-related corporate enterprise. Rather than restrict the dissemination of responsible, scientifically valid health information (as it does by preventing manufacturers from telling consumers about the disease-prevention effects of dietary fiber, beta-carotene, and even aspirin), the FDA would do well to establish a fair labeling system, letting consumers know that specific health claims or formulations *are* or *are not* approved by the FDA on the product labels themselves. An FDA disclaimer stating, for example, that "Published scientific evidence suggests that this product may help prevent [fill in the health claim here]; however, such evidence is currently inconclusive," would go a long way toward educating consumers, rather than restricting their access to scientifically sound information about the product.

Start Eating Smart Today

Eat Smart, Think Smart is the first book of its kind. It will show you how to feed your brain the smart nutrients it requires for maximum mental performance; just as important, it offers a nutritional blueprint to protect your brain against premature aging and all its consequences.

The book was written for apparently healthy and normal adults who want to provide their brains with the essential nutrients required for mental fitness. If you aspire to excellence, if you want to enjoy maximum mental performance at work and at play, if you want to protect your brain against premature aging, I urge you to read on without delay. Start building a better brain today.

Bon appétit!

Eat Smart, Think Smart

1

Smart Stuff for Your Brain:

How to Change Your Mind

How do smart people get smart? Is it all a matter of genetics? Luck? Or just plain hard work? Is there anything you can do to give yourself a mental, emotional, and creative boost—to spur your brain to its fullest potential?

You possess a unique set of biochemical attributes and environmental experiences that interact to produce the essence of who you are and, just as important, what you can become. Hard work alone is seldom enough to help you realize your full potential. The real achievers I've counseled all put in the necessary hours of work, study, and training to excel in their chosen professions. What separates the men from the boys, the women from the girls, the winners from the also-rans, is a biochemically charged flash of brilliance—that much-too-rare state of mind that you've undoubtedly already enjoyed at some point, if only briefly—in which you suddenly "see" the answers to difficult personal or professional problems or experience the kind of mental energy and creative insight that helps you improve your life and, perhaps, the lives of others.

It's those rare and fleeting instances of mental acuity, mood elevation, alertness, creativity, and lucidity that supply the often missing but vital 1 percent that makes the difference—the difference between mediocrity and excellence, the difference between graduating with honors or just graduating, the difference between job promotion or job stagnation.

I'm going to show you how you can literally change your mind. I will show you how to bathe your brain in smart nutrients that can boost mental and physical performance to new heights. I want to help you be the best you can be by showing you how to eat smart to think smart.

Everyone, from Socrates to Shakespeare, Newton to Einstein, Mozart to Paul McCartney, leapt to greatness with the help of the chemicals, made by their brains, from nutritional nuggets known as smart nutrients that they received naturally through the food they ate. With this book, you have an advantage they never had: By learning to control the amount and quality of smart nutrients through specially chosen foods and supplements, you can make smart nutrients work for you in the most focused possible way, raising your mental capacity, creativity and energy to higher levels than you ever dreamed possible. Although learning to derive maximum benefits from smart nutrients may not turn you into a genius, I can assure you that it will help you to become the mental and creative best you can be.

But smart nutrients can do more than increase your intelligence, memory, and mental energy. They can also boost your sex drive and prevent premature aging and senility. Smart substances can even burn off excess body fat, build muscle, help you get a good night's sleep, and elevate your mood to fight ordinary depression.

Information on smart nutrition is proliferating so quickly that few people can keep up with the thousands of articles published each month in medical and scientific journals, as well as in newspapers and popular magazines. *Eat Smart, Think Smart* will help you make sense of this highly technical and voluminous information and show you how to use it to improve your life. If you own a personal computer or have access to one, I'll show you how to keep abreast of future developments in smart nutrition. I'll also tell you how to use a personal computer to create, customize, and analyze maximum-performance diets for you and your family.

How to Use This Book

The Eat Smart, Think Smart plans are actually a series of separate smart-nutrient miniprograms that help you

- boost your mental energy, increase your memory, and fight depression
- burn off excess body fat
- promote antiaging strategies for the brain

- enhance your sex drive, orgasm, and mood
- get a good night's sleep
- build muscle with smart-nutrient alternatives to anabolic steroids
- learn about four important smart drugs

Each chapter provides a complete and separate smart-nutrient plan. You decide which plan addresses your specific needs. Some people may want to start with the chapter on mental energy and memory. Others may want to jump straight to the fat-burning chapter. Still others may want to discover the role that smart nutrients play in sexuality or how they can slow brain aging and prevent senility. I've made each miniplan easy to understand and follow.

For convenience and flexibility, you can choose one of three ways to enjoy smart nutrients: from nutritional supplements, from the smart foods that contain smart nutrients, or from a combination of the two. Many of my clients experiment to find the best of both worlds.

A note about the smart-nutrient supplements you'll learn about in these pages: Complete information about how to obtain every nutrient and vitamin supplement mentioned in this book can be found in Appendix I, which contains toll-free phone numbers and addresses of national and international suppliers and information on how to order the products by mail. In almost every case, premixed formulas can be purchased at your local health food store, vitamin shop, or pharmacy, but check Appendix I for the easiest and least expensive ways to obtain them if you can't find them locally. In Appendix II, you'll find information about special "smart" software that can turn your personal computer (PC) into a personal nutritionist that can find and track the smart nutrients in your whole family's diet. Appendix II contains a list of newsletters and magazines that regularly feature articles on smart drugs and nutrients as well as on related topics of life extension and health technology. In Appendix IV, you'll also learn how to use your PC to keep up with fast-breaking research information about smart nutrients and smart drugs by tapping into the power of on-line data-base services and electronic discussion groups with people all over the world. Appendix V is written for health care professionals and those readers with a background in the biomedical sciences. It contains the scientific rationale for the revolutionary Meltdown fat-burning formula discussed in Chapter 3. Recipes for delicious smart-food snacks and meals can be found in Chapter 9. Finally, the glossary of some of the less familiar terms and nutrients you'll read about in this book will give you an understanding of how smart nutrients can work for you.

But let's start with the basics. When we talk about the brain's "smart chemicals," what exactly are we talking about?

Your Brain's Own Smart Chemicals

When it comes to the gray matter of the brain, nothing is black and white. Scientists probably know more about the stars and planets of our galaxy than they do about the three-pound orb in our heads. But what is known about smart nutrients can help you accomplish a lot. The smart foods and nutrients that form the foundation of the Eat Smart, Think Smart plans can help your brain communicate with itself and the rest of your body by boosting the levels of its own smart chemicals.

How do smart nutrients make you smart? Your brain cells speak to one another by releasing neurotransmitters (made exclusively from smart nutrients) that chemically communicate a brief message to other cells in your brain and in the rest of your body. Neurotransmitters play a key role in controlling memory, mental energy, intelligence, sex drive, sleep, appetite, and mood every day. The six important brain neurotransmitters that you'll learn about at the end of this chapter and will read about throughout the book play a vital role in all areas of the Eat Smart, Think Smart plans because they are, in essence, your brain's own smart chemicals.

The smart nutrients and foods that form the foundation of the Eat Smart, Think Smart plans all contribute to the synthesis of these and other essential neurotransmitters. The smart nutrients—over forty of them are known already—are found in such foods as fish, fowl, beef, eggs, liver, beans, peas, lentils, and an array of ordinary garden vegetables, including carrots and broccoli. Some of these foods of animal origin contain such high levels of fat and cholesterol that I can't, in good conscience, recommend that you wolf them down indiscriminately to achieve maximum mental performance. Therefore, I'll show you how to get the smart nutrients you need from foods and supplements without running the risk of eating too much fat and cholesterol. Once you've learned how to feed your brain, I'll tell you about the newest smart nutrients and drinks and how they can protect your brain from premature aging and senility.

Your regular diet, if it meets the healthy nutritional guidelines I established in my first book, *Eat to Win,* already contains a modest mixture of smart nutrients. But I'll show you how to supplement your regular diet with the specific smart foods, special smart recipes (found in Chapter 9), and smart–nutrient formulas I'll tell you about in each of the other chapters.

Tennis champion Ivan Lendl learned the value of supplementing his smart nutrient–rich meals with formulas I've created to boost his alertness and energy on the court. Cher discovered how to start her long workdays on the movie set with my fat-burning smart breakfast beverage. Glenn Frey found that smart foods and nutrients could help stir the creative juices necessary to write and record beautiful and soulful songs. Boosting your brain's own smart chemicals can help you sustain your creative and mental energy just as dramatically.

Along with your newly acquired positive mental energy and creativity, you may begin to notice that a broader spectrum of ideas will present itself to you. You'll no longer solve problems solely by deciding between choices A, B, or C. Suddenly, something may occur to you that you hadn't previously considered (maybe A + B + C—what about D?). You'll focus on the solution to the problem you've been wrestling with in a new way, and you'll realize that until now, you've lacked this unique perspective. Whatever you need to accomplish will come easier and go more smoothly, with no hesitation, dread, or procrastination.

I know you think there's a catch, but there isn't. Because your body does not build up a tolerance to smart nutrients, you'll never have to take more to get the same effect. And when the smart nutrients wear off, they do so peacefully, so you don't "crash" or have a hangover. You'll feel nothing unusual—just the satisfaction of having done something worthwhile within the sixteen hours we call a day.

How Much of These Smart Nutrients Do You Need Each Day?

The amount of smart nutrients you need each day depends on a variety of factors: age (most neurotransmitter levels tend to decline as we grow older), illness (which depletes certain neurotransmitters), diet (some diets provide suboptimal levels of smart nutrients), drug use (tobacco, alcohol, recreational drugs, and prescription medications destroy smart nutrients) and stress (which depletes vitamins required to synthesize neurotransmitters). A number of published studies have helped define the safe and effective range of smart nutrient intake that can help you achieve maximum mental performance (your own intake of these nutrients may require some trial-and-error adjustment to optimize the dosage that works best for you).

A word about alcohol, tobacco, and other drugs: I discourage smoking and the excessive intake of alcohol because of their proved health risks, but I also know that we live in the real world, and some of you do smoke and drink. The good news is that the antioxidant, antiaging smart nutrients I'll tell you about can help to counteract the negative effects of smoking, drinking, and aging on the brain. Although these habits will never be good for you, if you do smoke and drink, you'll be able to keep yourself in better health with smart nutrients than you could without them.

Crossing the Blood-Brain Barrier

Mother Nature designed an excellent fortress—the blood-brain barrier (BBB)—to protect the brain from the onslaught of chemicals we take into our bodies each day. The BBB (actually a series of small blood vessels and special cells that support and nourish brain neurons called glial cells) controls, to a certain extent, the entry of smart nutrients and smart drugs into your brain. This is beneficial because too much of anything, even water and air, can be harmful.

Several decades ago, when researchers discovered that the BBB controlled the flow into the brain of raw materials that are necessary for synthesizing neurotransmitters, they also discovered that by increasing the ratio of one smart nutrient to the others (in this case, amino acids), they could saturate the BBB's transport mechanisms that lock on to that specific nutrient and carry it into the brain. The result was that they could get more of one smart nutrient into the brain simply by overfeeding it relative to all others.

Scientists also discovered that brain neurotransmitter levels could be increased by a *single meal*. For example, protein-rich foods, such as chicken, turkey, and seafood, can boost the levels of norepinephrine in the brain, with a subsequent improvement in alertness. In contrast, a meal rich in carbohydrates will increase the levels of serotonin in the brain, leading to relaxation, satiety, and even sleep.

Vitamins are also required for promoting the synthesis of brain neurotransmitters, although they do not compete with each other for entry into the brain as amino acids do (for example, the brain has its own special vitamin C pump to ensure an abundant supply of this important smart nutrient; other vitamins are "carried" into the brain by special carrier-molecules). The brain uses vitamin B_3 and vitamin B_6 to convert the amino acid L-tryptophan into the mood- and sleep-regulating neurotransmitter serotonin. Vitamins B_3, B_6, C, and folic acid and the minerals copper, iron, and zinc are all needed to transform the amino acids L-phenylalanine and L-tyrosine into dopamine and norepinephrine. Vitamins B_1, B_5, B_6, and C and the minerals zinc and calcium are required for the production of acetylcholine.

We'll never know how much acetylcholine pulsed through Albert Einstein's brain when he developed his theory of relativity, just as we'll never find out how much norepinephrine bathed the brain of the composer Ludwig van Beethoven, when he wrote his Fifth Symphony. One thing I do know: Smart nutrients offer a real chance to help us be the best we can be. They protect the brain from the ravages of aging while supplying it with the very nutrients that every great mind in history has relied upon to achieve maximum mental performance.

Your Brain's Super-Six Neurotransmitters

Now let's find out exactly what your brain's own "smart chemicals" are.

Your body manufactures neurotransmitters (the brain's smart chemicals that allow you to think, feel, perform, and look your best) from nutrients in foods we eat each day. Intelligence, memory, antiaging, sexuality, sleep, mood elevation, and weight loss all depend, to a large extent, on providing the body with the raw materials that the brain uses to manufacture key neurotransmitters. Almost all the major neurotransmitters either are or are made from amino acids, the building blocks of protein. Upon digestion, our bodies break down whole protein (from plant and animal foods) into hundreds of thousands of amino acids. From there, the amino acids are carried in the blood to various organs, including muscles (for growth, maintenance, and energy) and the brain (for synthesizing neurotransmitters).

The following is a list of six key neurotransmitters that can help you achieve maximum mental performance each day, followed by a precise description of how each of them works:

- Acetylcholine
- Norepinephrine
- Dopamine
- Serotonin
- L-glutamate
- GABA (gamma-aminobutyric acid)

ACETYLCHOLINE. Acetylcholine is the most abundant neurotransmitter in the body and is the primary neurotransmitter between neurons and muscles. It helps the body perform a variety of "housekeeping" functions. The stomach, spleen, bladder, liver, sweat glands, blood vessels, and heart are just some of the organs that this neurotransmitter partially controls. Unlike most other neurotransmitters, such as GABA and serotonin, which can be used to manage specific conditions, such as aggressive behavior and insomnia, respectively, acetylcholine cannot be used as a supplement in and of itself because of its diffuseness of action (and its rapid breakdown). Still, the body's synthesis of acetylcholine is vital because of that neurotransmitter's role in motor behavior (muscular movement) and memory.

Low levels of acetylcholine can contribute to the lack of concentration and forgetfulness and may cause you to be a light sleeper. Outside the brain, acetylcholine plays an essential role in keeping mucous membranes properly moistened.

The body synthesizes the neurotransmitter acetylcholine from the smart nutrients choline, lecithin, and DMAE and ancillary nutrient cofactors, such as vitamins C, B_1, B_5, and B_6, along with the minerals zinc and calcium. Acetylcholine helps control muscle tone, learning, and primitive drives and emotions. It also controls the release of the pituitary hormone vasopressin, which is involved in learning and in the regulation of urine output.

NOREPINEPHRINE. Norepinephrine stimulates the release of stored body fat and helps control the release of endocrine hormones, which help regulate fertility, sex drive, appetite, and metabolism. It is also intimately involved in boosting learning and memory. Norepinephrine influences sleep and wake patterns and helps maintain the normal function of the immune system. Low levels of norepinephrine can lead to depression. Norepinephrine is synthesized from two amino acids—L-phenylalanine and L-tyrosine (found in large amounts in animal foods, such as chicken, turkey, seafood, and beef)—and several vitamins and minerals, including vitamin C, B_3, B_6, and copper.

DOPAMINE. Dopamine affects the movement of muscles, the growth and repair of tissues, the sex drive, and the functioning of the immune system. It also stimulates the pituitary gland to secrete growth hormone, which builds muscle, burns fat, and promotes healing and a healthy immune system. Low levels of dopamine can lead to depression and Parkinson's disease (a gradual but fatal diminution of muscular control), whereas high levels have been linked to schizophrenia. Dopamine is chemically related to norepinephrine and L-dopa (a prescription drug used to treat Parkinson's disease) and, like norepinephrine, is synthesized from the amino acids L-phenylalanine and L-tyrosine.

SEROTONIN. Serotonin is found in high concentrations in blood platelets, the gastrointestinal tract, and certain regions of the brain. It plays an important role in blood clotting, stimulating a strong heart beat, initiating sleep, fighting depression (prescription drugs that treat depression raise the brain's levels of serotonin) and causing migraine headaches in susceptible individuals (because of its ability to constrict blood vessels or cause them to spasm). Serotonin is synthesized from the amino acid L-tryptophan. Serotonin (and, therefore, L-tryptophan) also serves as a precursor for the pineal hormone melatonin, which helps regulate the body's clock.

L-GLUTAMATE. The brain and central nervous system contain high concentrations of the amino acid L-glutamate, which exerts powerful excitatory (as well as some inhibitory) effects on memory neurons in almost every area of the central nervous system. Low brain levels of L-glutamate can lead to decreased mental and physical performance. Much research still needs to be done to delineate its manifold functions and its role in boosting maximum mental performance.

GABA. One of the most well-researched inhibitory neurotransmitters, GABA (gamma-aminobutyric acid) plays an important role in relaxation, sedation, and sleep. Many prescription medications rely on the brain's GABA-sensitive system (a complex of cell membrane receptors and related nerves that use GABA as a chemical messenger) to work. Valium and Librium, two of the most often-prescribed muscle relaxants and sedatives, attach to GABA-type receptors to achieve their sedative action. Many smart drugs are based on the molecular structure of GABA, although they appear to affect the brain in entirely different ways. GABA is available as an over-the-counter nutritional supplement.

These are just six of over fifty neurotransmitters your brain uses each day, but they are six of the most important chemicals that you can boost using the smart nutrients that form the core of the Eat Smart, Think Smart series of miniplans. Ultimately, they're what we want to boost to optimal levels so we can enjoy their maximum benefits.

Let's learn how to do that right now. You're about to give your brain a wake-up call—and much more.

An Overview of Smart Nutrition

Anti-Aging

- Coenzyme Q10
- Ascorbyl Palmitate
- PPQ
- Vitamin C
- Choline
- α-Tocopherol
- DMAE
- Beta-Carotene
- Vitamin B-Complex
- Inositol
- Selenium
- n-Acetyl Cysteine
- Gingko Biloba
- PABA
- L-Glutathione
- Green Tea

Creativity

- Green Tea
- Choline
- DMAE
- Gingko Biloba
- D-Glucose
- Vitamin B-Complex
- Pantothenic Acid
- Vitamin C
- Zinc

Memory and Learning

- DMAE
- Choline
- n-Acetyl Carnitine
- L-Tyrosine
- Vitamin B12
- Boron
- Pantothenic Acid
- Gingko Biloba
- Green Tea
- Pyridoxine
- Vitamin C
- Vitamin E
- Zinc

Energy

- Coenzyme Q$_{10}$
- Ascorbyl Palmitate
- Vitamin C
- Vitamin B-Complex
- Pantothenic Acid
- D-Glucose
- Ginkgo Biloba
- L-Carnitine
- DMAE
- L-Leucine
- K$^+$ / Mg^{++} Phosphate
- L-Tyrosine

Sleep

- L-Tryptophan
- Niacinamide
- Inositol
- GABA
- Pyridoxine

Weight Loss

- Green Tea
- Ma Huang
- L-Carnitine
- Choline
- K$^+$ / Mg^{++} Phosphate
- White Willow Bark
- Chromium Picolinate

Sexuality

- α-Tocopherol
- Choline
- Vitamin C
- Lecithin
- L-Tyrosine
- Pyridoxine
- Zinc

Anabolics

- L-Arginine
- L-Ornithine
- Chromium Picolinate
- Boron
- L-Tryptophan
- L-Leucine
- Ma Huang (Ephedra)

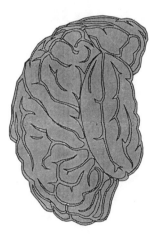

2

Wake Up Your Brain with Mind-Fitness Nutrients

Imagine that you're jogging around the reservoir in Central Park, New York City. A group of your less-active friends are sitting on a nearby bench watching you. They wave each time you pass, but choose not to get up and join you. You are all enjoying the weather and vistas of the city's skyline, but only one of you is really accomplishing anything. They're living for the moment while you're living for future days, as well as today.

Now picture the same kind of scenario in a mental milieu because mind fitness can be as exhilarating as is physical fitness. Think about the possibilities of getting more out of a learning experience than those around you: having material leap off the page with meaning and possibility when you read and remembering the meaning, details, and all you've learned, days or weeks later.

Certain people seem to be able to do this naturally. It's as if they have the *Cliff Notes* to life. We all probably know people who have seemingly boundless mental energy that allows them to learn and recall facts with relative ease and to squeeze more out of an hour's work than most of us accomplish in a day. These people enjoy the cerebral vitality and stamina that can come only from their brain's own smart chemicals—chemicals that your brain could probably use more of.

If you're a mental couch potato, don't despair. Mind-fitness nutrients will get you off the couch and onto the fast track of success and achievement. Maximum mental performers use their brains more because mind-fitness nutrients give their brains the mental energy to do so.

You may be familiar with the expression "hitting the wall," which marathon runners use to denote a state of physical exhaustion characterized by the lack of energy, muscle cramps, and debilitating fatigue. Even though you may never consider running twenty-six miles, you may have already run smack into another kind of wall—a mental wall that can cause mental burnout or just the lack of fresh and exciting ideas.

Over a decade ago, I showed world-class marathon runners how to avoid hitting the wall by following a diet that is high in complex carbohydrates, low in fat, and moderate in protein. When I first started telling coaches, trainers, and team physicians about my discoveries, few listened. Fortunately, a handful of champion athletes did, and today, my dietary advice is followed by millions of people the world over.

Now, I'm going to show you a new way to use smart nutrients to break through mental walls that can bring productivity and creativity to a grinding halt, costing you time and money each day. Just as marathon runners and other endurance athletes use my dietary advice to avoid hitting the wall, you, too, can use my smart-nutrient formulas and recipes to become a mental athlete.

This chapter covers a good deal of territory. First, you'll learn what the brain's basic food is and how to time your meals so your brain will get as much of this basic fuel as possible. Then you'll get a shopping list of the basic smart nutrients that affect memory, mental energy, and mood elevation, along with guidelines about recommended dosages and the foods in which the smart nutrients are most commonly found. Next, you'll find a list of foods from which you can choose combinations that will achieve many of the same effects you get from the smart-nutrient supplement formulas I'll give you later on—you'll learn how to construct an overall mental wake-up diet to act as a good smart-food base for the mental fine-tuning you may want to do with supplements later on. Finally, I'll tell you about a super choline cocktail that is designed to lift your mental energy, acuity, and focus. This smart drink will help increase your mental energy and focus right away, supply your brain with nutrients that facilitate memory, and elevate your mood and fight depression and hence create an overall climate for good mental functioning. As with all the formulas in this book, I'll tell you how to purchase this choline cocktail ready made or how to make it yourself with widely available nutritional supplements that you mix with your favorite beverage. You'll learn that you can boost your brain power through food and fast-acting smart drinks. You've got a lot of mental energy options.

But first—what do our brains want to "eat"?

To Boost Your Brain, Reach for Protein First

You can actually control your own level of mental performance—or relaxation—by choosing the right combination of foods that contain smart nutrients.

Two amino acids compete with one another to control the way your brain works. One is L-tyrosine, which your brain uses to synthesize the neurotransmitters norepinephrine and dopamine, both of which are critical to lucid, swift thinking; long-term memory; and feelings of alertness and stability. The other is L-tryptophan, which the brain uses to make the neurotransmitter serotonin, which is responsible for slowing down reaction time, imparting satiety after a meal, and inducing sleep. L-tyrosine, found in protein-rich foods like meat, poultry, seafood, beans, tofu, and lentils, thus serves as a nutritional stimulant to the brain, whereas L-tryptophan, found in such foods as bananas, sunflower seeds, and milk (and whose effects are augmented when consumed with carbohydrate-rich foods), behaves as a mental downer.

If L-tyrosine gets into your brain ahead of L-tryptophan, it will prime your brain to function at maximum performance levels all day (or all night, depending upon when you eat the meal or snack). But if L-tryptophan reaches the brain first, it will stimulate the production of serotonin, and your mental performance will ebb and your brain will begin to shut down, even in the middle of the day.

Where do you get these amino acids, and how do you get them into your brain? The answers to these two questions reveal how easy it is to begin a program of mental fitness and how you can exert a good measure of control over your own levels of mental performance, memory, relaxation, and even depression.

Judith Wurtman, Ph.D., a researcher at the Massachusetts Institute of Technology (MIT) advises that when you want the mental lift from L-tyrosine, you should eat the protein portion of a meal (turkey or shrimp, for example) before you take a single bite of any food that contains carbohydrates (the same applies to beverages). I recommend 100 grams (3½ ounces) of animal protein, such as a boneless chicken breast or a small can of water-packed tuna fish. Vegetarians can use textured vegetable protein (TVP), tofu, or legumes (such as beans, peas, or lentils) in place of meat to get their L-tyrosine.

Animal and vegetable protein is chock-full of L-tyrosine, but contains only modest amounts of L-tryptophan. Thus, L-tyrosine will crowd-out L-tryptophan and cross the BBB in greater amounts. Your brain will wake up as a result.

Another reason that L-tyrosine prevails over L-tryptophan is that L-tryptophan also needs carbohydrates to get into the brain. Several ounces of protein-rich food, such as turkey, will send plenty of L-tyrosine to your brain; L-tryptophan, however, cannot readily cross the BBB until you eat the carbohydrate-rich foods—breads, pastas, and vegetables— you left on your plate (carbohydrates stimulate the release of insulin, which drives other competing amino acids into muscles, leaving L-tryptophan to cross the BBB into the brain unopposed).

Do you sometimes feel lethargic after lunch? One of the most common complaints I hear is, "By mid-afternoon, I can't concentrate very well. I could use more energy!" Actually, the type of energy most people want is *mental* energy, exactly the kind you'll get from a high-protein power lunch (and the choline "cocktail" I'll tell you about shortly). If you hold off on the pasta until dinner, you'll enjoy peak mental energy when you need it most—during the workday—and benefit from the relaxation effects of L-tryptophan in the evening, when it's time to wind down, relax, and fall asleep.

L-tyrosine's ability to rev up your brain may even help overcome stress and depression. The U.S. Army discovered that L-tyrosine was able to counter the effects of mental stress and depression on the performance of soldiers. Two dozen soldiers were tested with and without supplemental L-tyrosine before a stressful maneuver, half of them receiving L-tyrosine and half of them receiving a placebo, an inert substance free of L-tyrosine. The stressful operation was repeated again, this time so that those who received the placebo got L-tyrosine and those who received L-tyrosine the first time got the placebo.

During the two maneuvers, the soldiers were tested to determine their ability to perform military tasks that required clear thinking and quick decisions. The result was that those who normally experienced stress or depression that adversely affected their thinking and performance (as well as headaches, fatigue, and muddled thinking) found that L-tyrosine reduced their stress and depression while improving their performance. It is interesting that soldiers who normally experienced little, if any, stress or depression found that L-tyrosine did not make much difference in their performance. This finding may imply that people who consume enough

L-tyrosine-rich foods, such as chicken, turkey, and seafood, won't enjoy the same degree of brain stimulation from L-tyrosine supplements as will those who have not ingested optimal amounts of this smart amino acid.

Glucose: The Primary Mental-Energy Nutrient

Even though carbohydrates help relax the brain, they are necessary for maximum mental performance. If consumption is *properly timed,* carbohydrate-rich foods, such as pasta, bread, legumes, cereals, grains, fruits, and vegetables, can boost the brain's energy levels.

Carbohydrates—combinations of carbon, oxygen, and hydrogen molecules that are abundant in foods that are high in starch and sugar—are quickly broken down by the body into the brain's most important food: glucose, a basic sugar found throughout nature. Carbohydrates enhance mental performance because your brain is a glucose addict. Glucose is the "drug" your brain craves, every second of every day. It supplies your brain with the most basic type of energy it needs to do just about everything brains do: think, remember, solve problems, and control the rest of the body.

Foods that are rich in complex carbohydrates, such as whole grains, brown rice, unrefined cereals and flour, and vegetables and fruits, provide your brain with a steady supply of glucose (a glycemic index, or measure of the degree to which foods raise levels of blood sugar, indicates which foods to pick: Those with a lower glycemic rating provide the brain with glucose at a steadier rate and thus are preferable to foods with a high glycemic rating; see Chart 2.1).

That's why a diet that includes a generous supply of complex carbohydrates (60–80 percent of daily kilocalories) constitutes the dietary foundation for achieving maximum mental energy. "Simple" carbohydrates, such as refined sugar and flour (or foods made primarily from refined sugar and flour), give your body and brain a quick glucose blast, followed by a crash. Although the brain gets flooded for a short period by glucose, it is just as suddenly deprived of it and quickly craves more—hence the common experience of a sugar "hangover." In general, most complex carbohydrates are preferable because of their time-release properties: They give you a steadier and longer-term flow of glucose and thus more mental and physical energy.

My research has shown that a daily intake of 300–400 grams per day of complex carbohydrates from all food sources provides enough basic brain fuel to start you on the road to maximum mental performance. This amount translates into about 1,200–1,600 kilocalories each day (out of a

CHART 2.1

Index of Glycemic (Blood Sugar–Increasing) Ratings of Selected Foods

The following numbers indicate the relative ability of selected foods to raise blood sugar levels. Foods with higher numbers (with glucose being arbitrarily set at the highest, 100) raise blood sugar the quickest.

Glucose	100
Baked potato	98
Carrots	92
Honey	87
White rice	72
Wheat bread	72
White bread	69
Brown rice	66
Banana	62
Sucrose (table sugar)	59
Spaghetti	50
Orange juice	46
Grapes	45
Apples	39
Yogurt	36
Whole milk	34
Skim milk	32
Grapefruit	26
Red cherries	23
Fructose	20

total of about 1,800–2,200 kilocalories per day, on average) from whole-grain breads, cereals, grains, fruits, and vegetables.

Just as with protein, however, *when* you eat carbohydrates is critical to how your brain will respond. Timing is everything. As you can see from Chart 2.2, you should use protein-rich foods to help you start your day and whenever you need to boost alertness; add complex carbohydrate-rich foods as snacks or side dishes to maintain glucose levels in the brain, and use carbohydrates as a main course when you want to calm your brain (at dinner or late in the evening, for example).

Consuming protein-rich foods and timing your intake of complex carbohydrates to control mental energy marks the first step to achieving maximum mental performance. The next step requires the use of high-energy smart-nutrient supplements that work by supplying your brain with the additional raw materials it needs to help you work at peak performance levels throughout the day and evening, if necessary.

CHART 2.2

Smart Times for Smart Foods

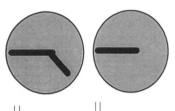 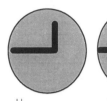 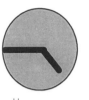

Use this chart to help you maximize mental energy throughout the day and evening; in general, you should start the day with a mixture of foods rich in protein and complex carbohydrates; lunch should contain a protein-rich entrée; midday snacks should supply carbo-fuel for your brain; dinner should include choline-rich foods, such as seafood or legumes; bedtime snacks should contain a rich supply of tryptophan.

Breakfast

Begin the day with a mixture of protein and complex carbohydrates: low-fat milk with whole-grain cereal and fresh fruit.

Lunch

To renew mental energy for the afternoon, have a salad with low-fat dressing, shrimp cocktail, or chicken breast (remove skin) and fresh fruit for dessert.

Afternoon Snack

Use the midday snack to supply your brain with carbohydrates. Choose fresh fruit or low-fat crackers with six ounces of fruit juice or vegetable juice cocktail.

Dinner

Start the evening with complex carbohydrates—baked potato or corn—as a side dish; choose a choline-rich entrée, such as lentil soup or fish; and finish with a low-fat frozen yogurt dessert.

Bedtime Snack

Relax your brain and prepare for a good night's sleep with bananas or banana custard or enjoy the "Lights Out" toddy (see Chapter 9).

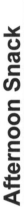 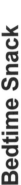

If your brain is sluggish, smart nutrients, such as choline, will help reestablish a more normal level of operation. Others, such as green tea (a source of methyl xanthines, including caffeine, and antioxidants called polyphenols), ginkgo biloba (an herbal brain-metabolism booster), and DMAE (a source of choline that can be stored in brain neurons), act as brain stimulants. Unlike amphetamines and other potentially harmful stimulants, smart nutrients are nonaddicting (although caffeine may be addicting for some people), and they won't let you crash or suffer a drug hangover.

Mind-fitness nutrients also seem to give people a sense of heightened creativity, inventiveness, and artistry. Although it's difficult, if not impossible, to document scientifically the increased creativity that many people experience with mind-fitness nutrients, the fact is that many people *do* feel more creative and productive as a result of them. See for yourself; you'll enjoy the same benefits.

A Shopping List of Smart Nutrients

You can use mind-fitness nutrients to rejuvenate sluggish mental performance, to elevate your mood, and to think more clearly, especially when you face a demanding work or study schedule. In addition, these nutrients improve the blood supply to the brain and help protect it from damage by free radicals. Research studies have found that mind-fitness nutrients can actually extend the life span of laboratory animals 30–50 percent.

Here is an inventory of mind-fitness nutrients that can help rev up your brain to its maximum performance levels. I've listed dosages that are commonly used in most commercially available smart-nutrient products, in case you want to take one or another of them separately to judge their effectiveness for yourself. You'll see that many of the following nutrients appear in the "choline cocktail" formula for mental energy and memory that appears right after this list.

GINKGO BILOBA. Ginkgo biloba is extracted from the leaves of the oldest-known surviving species of tree, the ginkgo tree. Chinese physicians have used ginkgo-leaf extract for thousands of years to boost cerebral metabolism, improve blood flow to the brain, and augment mental alertness. Dozens of published studies on humans have revealed that gingko increases brain metabolism by promoting the synthesis of ATP (adenosine triphosphate—the primary energy-producing molecule in the body), improving the brain's ability to metabolize glucose, its primary fuel, and helping to prevent blood clotting in the brain's arteries. Ginkgo also acts as an antioxidant smart nutrient and has been shown to improve short-term memory in the elderly. It increases the brain's alpha electrical rhythms, associated with alertness, and decreases the brain's theta rhythms, associated with lack of attention and an unfocused state of mind. It is available either as a powder in capsules or in liquid form.

Dosage commonly used: Most published studies have used ginkgo extract standardized to a 24 percent concentration (look for this number on the package label and accept no less). At this strength, the typical dosage is 120–150 mg per day, divided into three equal doses.

CAFFEINE. Caffeine (and related methyl-xanthine compounds) is probably the best known mind-fitness nutrient in the United States. Millions of coffee- and tea lovers may be addicted not so much to the stimulant properties of caffeine, but to the paradoxical calming effect it has on many people. Coffee actually contains several opiate-related compounds that exert a mild heroinlike effect on the brain. These compounds are found in decaffeinated coffee as well. Caffeine helps improve typing skills (the number of error-free typed words per minute), mental alertness, energy, and the ability to do work even when fatigued (caffeine improves mental stamina by stimulating the release of norepinephrine in the brain).

Dosage commonly used: Most published research indicates that apparently healthy people can consume up to 200 mg per day (the approximate amount in two cups of brewed coffee) without any adverse health effects. Green tea, generally sold in health food stores, contains about 100 mg of caffeine per serving and potent antioxidant smart nutrients, called polyphenols, that recent research has shown may protect against damage to arteries that can lead to heart attack and stroke.

VITAMIN B$_1$ (THIAMIN) AND B$_2$ (RIBOFLAVIN). These B vitamins help control energy production from glucose in the brain and the nervous system. They assist in the formation of the fatty acids that lend structural integrity to membranes of nerve cells (neurons) and participate in the synthesis of the memory-related brain neurotransmitter acetylcholine. Eating raw fish or raw eggs or chronic alcohol consumption can destroy vitamin B$_1$; vitamin B$_2$ is destroyed by light and cooking.

Dosage commonly used: Most high-potency vitamin formulas on the market contain 10 to 50 mg each of thiamin and riboflavin.

VITAMIN B$_3$ (NIACINAMIDE). A deficiency of this vitamin leads to a condition known as pellagra, characterized by malfunctioning of the nervous system, gastrointestinal disturbances (indigestion, anorexia), and skin inflammation. Your brain and nervous system require optimal amounts of niacinamide to perform at maximum levels (the body can also convert the amino acid L-tryptophan into niacin; some authorities believe that up to two-thirds of the body's daily requirement can be satisfied by L-tryptophan).

Dosage commonly used: Most brain formulas contain 25–125 mg per day of niacinamide. Large doses of another form of vitamin B_3, niacin (also called nicotinic acid), have been used in the medical treatment of elevated blood cholesterol and triglycerides. Since pure niacin causes skin flushing and burning and may aggravate health problems, including stomach ulcers, diabetes mellitus, and liver disease, you should use pure niacin *only when advised to do so by your physician.*

VITAMIN B_5. Known as pantothenic acid (because it occurs in foods of both plant and animal origin), this vitamin participates in the synthesis of the brain neurotransmitter acetylcholine.

VITAMIN B_6. Also called pyridoxine, this vitamin promotes maximum mental performance by aiding in the transport and metabolism of the amino acids used by the brain to manufacture neurotransmitters involved in mental energy and memory. A deficiency of vitamin B_6 can lead to brain-wave abnormalities and malfunctioning of the nervous system. Chronic megadoses of this vitamin (2 to 6 grams per day) that are used to treat carpal tunnel syndrome have led, in a few cases, to vitamin toxicity (peripheral neuropathy), which disappeared once the dosage of B_6 was reduced.

Dosage commonly used: Most high-potency multivitamin formulas supply 10 to 75 mg of vitamin B_6 per day. Certain conditions, such as pregnancy; the use of oral contraceptives; and increased protein intake can increase your need for vitamin B_6.

People taking L-dopa for Parkinson's disease should not take supplemental vitamin B_6 because it can diminish the effects of L-dopa in the brain. Vitamin B_6 can cause nerve problems when used in doses above 400 mg per day for long periods of time. Check with a physician before using megadoses of vitamin B_6.

CHOLINE AND LECITHIN. Choline and phosphatidyl choline (popularly known as lecithin) increase the brain's synthesis of acetylcholine, a neurotransmitter involved in memory, learning, and mental alertness. Choline and lecithin supplements come in a variety of forms: liquid choline (usually as choline chloride), encapsulated choline (as choline bitartrate), and lecithin granules (look for lecithin products that contain at least 55 percent phosphatidyl choline). Other mind-fitness nutrients, such as vitamin B_{12} and glutathione, can substitute for many of choline's biochemical functions, but only choline; lecithin; and a functionally related compound, DMAE (see next listing), can appreciably boost levels of acetylcholine in the brain. Peanuts, wheat germ, ham, trout, and calf's liver are rich sources of lecithin; brussels sprouts, oatmeal, soybeans, cabbage, cauliflower, kale, spinach, carrots, lettuce, and potatoes also contain appreciable amounts of choline chloride.

Dosage commonly used: Most memory-boosting supplement formulas on the market (such as Twin Lab's Choline Cocktail) contain 1,500 mg of choline chloride or choline bitartrate (choline chloride is also available in liquid form). Lecithin (phosphatidyl choline) is marketed in capsules, granules, liquids, and baked goods. Look for products that contain at least 55 percent lecithin by weight, as noted on the package labels. Choline, unlike amino acids, does not have to be taken on an empty stomach because no known nutrient competes with it for absorption.

Persons with gastric ulcers or a history of ulcers should use choline supplements only with consent of a physician; choline may increase stomach acid production; choline supplements should not be used by persons with Parkinson's disease or by those who are taking prescription anticholinergic drugs.

DMAE (DIMETHYLAMINOETHANOL). Like choline and lecithin, DMAE can increase the brain's production of acetylcholine. Recent studies have shown that DMAE can elevate mood, improve memory and learning, and even extend the life span of laboratory animals. Although DMAE is a nutrient found in seafood, such as sardines and anchovies, some smart-nutrient formulas call for 100–500 mg, which requires the use of a DMAE supplement (available as a liquid or a powder). DMAE has been used to treat learning disorders in children who are diagnosed as underachievers, those with shortened attention spans, or those who are hyperactive. The brain-stimulant effect of DMAE develops slowly over a period of weeks, with no druglike letdown when discontinued. Published studies have noted that DMAE in low doses can, ironically, be used to induce sleep.

Dosage commonly used: DMAE is a volatile compound that should be stored in a dark, cool place. It is available in bulk powder form, liquid, and capsules. Smart-nutrient users generally start with low doses of DMAE (100 mg per day) with a gradual buildup to 500 mg per day. Overdosage (more than 500 mg per day in some cases) can cause insomnia, headaches, and muscle tension. People with epilepsy should be monitored by a physician if they use DMAE. Those who suffer from manic-depressive illness should avoid taking DMAE because it can intensify the depressive phase.

VITAMIN C. The brain and central nervous system contain a high concentration of vitamin C. Brain cells have a high content of unsaturated fat, which makes them susceptible to oxidation and damage from toxic atoms or molecules called free radicals. Thus, high levels of vitamin C are required to prevent brain damage and premature aging. Published studies have shown that students with higher vitamin C levels in their blood scored better on IQ tests than did those with lower vitamin C levels. Vitamin C is required for the synthesis of acetylcholine and norepinephrine.

Dosage commonly used: Many health professionals recommend vitamin C intakes far above the RDA of 60 mg. Many brain formulas contain 500 mg to 1,000 mg of some form of vitamin C (the less acidic form, calcium ascorbate, is widely available for people with sensitive stomachs; the fat-soluble form, ascorbyl palmitate, is found in "brain formulas" on the market and is available as a nutritional supplement).

COENZYME Q_{10}. CoQ_{10} helps create brain energy in the form of ATP, and it serves as a free-radical scavenger that protects the brain's cell membranes. Tissue concentrations of CoQ_{10} are depleted under a variety of conditions, including stress, various illnesses, exposure to cold, drug use, and physical activity. Seafood is a rich source of CoQ_{10}, with white albacore tuna (the kind packed with spring water in cans) containing the highest amount.

Dosage commonly used: No one has yet determined the amount of CoQ_{10} needed for optimal health (this amount will vary from individual to individual), but published research reveals that dosages in the range of 10–90 mg per day are safe and effective.

VITAMIN B_{12} AND FOLIC ACID. I've lumped these two vitamins together because of their similar functions. Vitamin B_{12} is unusual in that the only source in nature is synthesis by microorganisms, that is, the vitamin is not found in plants except when contaminated by microbes. (Intestinal bacteria can synthesize a small amount of vitamin B_{12}, but animals, including humans, cannot get enough from their own bacteria and so must obtain it through the diet. The vitamin B_{12} that you got from the steak you ate last night originally came from the bacteria that lived in the feed eaten by the steer.) The common food sources of vitamin B_{12} are meat; fish (including clams, oysters, crab, salmon, and sardines); poultry; and, to a lesser extent, milk products, such as nonfat dry milk. Vitamin B_{12} is required for the transportation and storage of folic acid. It also helps regulate the metabolism of carbohydrates and proteins in the brain and the synthesis of myelin in the nerves (myelin is the protective fatty sheath surrounding nerve branches) and is involved, indirectly, in making choline available for the synthesis of neurotransmitters.

Folic acid is required for the synthesis of memory molecules (such as ribonucleic acid, or RNA) in the brain. It also helps control protein metabolism in the brain (involving at least two neurotransmitters, glutamic acid and glycine), and plays an essential role in the development of the nervous system in the fetus. Common food sources of folic acid include green, leafy vegetables, such as lettuce, spinach, kale, and collard greens; folic acid is also present in fresh fruits. Vitamin B_6, another mind-fitness nutrient discussed previously, is intimately involved in the metabolic roles played by vitamin B_{12} and folic acid.

Dosage commonly used: High-potency multiple vitamin–mineral supplements generally supply 500–1,000 mcg of vitamin B_{12} and 100–800 mcg of folic acid. Recent research has shown that oral vitamin B_{12} supplements are absorbed well even by elderly people, who may have an impaired ability to absorb this vitamin.

CHROMIUM PICOLINATE. This special form of the mineral chromium was developed and patented by scientists at the U.S. Department of Agriculture. Chromium helps the hormone insulin remove carbohydrates from the blood and get them into brain cells, where they can be metabolized for energy. Chromium picolinate seems to work more efficiently than does ordinary chromium and has been shown to have anabolic, or muscle-building, effects in people who take it and exercise regularly.

Dosage commonly used: Recently published studies have used 200 mcg per day for women. Some experts believe that weight lifters and other athletes of both sexes may need up to 400 mcg per day. Chromium picolinate is available in "smart" drinks, high-potency multiple vitamin–mineral formulas, and in 200 mcg capsules.

How to Eat Smart: Finding Smart Nutrients in Foods

For those who literally want to eat smart nutrients instead of get them from a bottle, I've listed selected smart foods that will supply your brain with the essential raw materials it needs for maximum mental performance. But before I give you lists of smart foods that contain substantial nutrition in addition to a rich supply of mind-fitness nutrients, you need to learn a little about how to mix them for the best effects.

Timing and the proper selection of foods are critical: To bathe your brain in the raw materials it needs to function properly, you'll need to select smart foods that contain a rich supply of specific amino acids and eat them at the right time.

L-tyrosine is the primary amino acid you need to boost brain levels of dopamine and norepinephrine, essential for mental energy, memory function, and even sex drive. Select smart-food combinations that are rich in this amino acid (and in L-phenylalanine) from the list presented here. If you need more mental energy at any point in the day, consume them *alone* to promote maximum absorption across the BBB.

Consume phenylalanine + tyrosine-rich foods about two hours after your previous meal and at least one hour before your next meal. Choline-rich foods can be eaten at any time, since choline's absorption is not compromised by other nutrients.

Here are a few examples of foods that make healthy and delicious food combinations for increasing mental energy and performance (the recipes for items in bold type can be found in Chapter 9).

- 1 cup of dry-roasted soybeans and ½ cup of low-fat cottage cheese
- surf and turf: 3 ounces of lobster plus 3 ounces of sirloin
- 1 cup of **Pea, Bean, and Lentil soup** and 3 ounces of tuna salad
- egg-white omelet with 2 ounces of diced ham
- 4 ounces of poached salmon with 2 ounces of **Herb Yogurt Dressing**
- **Italian-Style Sole** (one serving)
- **Mexican Snapper** (one serving)
- 3 ounces of chicken- or turkey-breast salad with low-fat dressing

Creating Your Own Smart Drink: The Super "Choline Cocktail"

I've given this choline cocktail to many of my clients who needed mental energy, memory enhancement, and antioxidant protection against age-accelerating free radicals.

I created the prototype for my choline cocktail in Cher's kitchen blender to help her perform at peak levels on movie sets, during recording sessions, and for enhanced mind fitness during a worldwide promotional tour for her movie *Mask* (for which she won the Best Actress award at the Cannes

Film Festival). Since then, I have modified it to conform to the latest discoveries in smart nutrition. You can make it in your own kitchen blender from its component nutrients, all of which are available in your local health food store. For convenience, you can also purchase the cocktail ready made (presweetened with NutraSweet or with sugar). At this time, the only similar version of my choline cocktail formula available nationally in health food stores is Twin Lab's Choline Cocktail, but many other companies' choline formulations are available by mail order (see Appendix I for addresses and telephone numbers).

Super Choline Cocktail Recipe

1,500 mg choline
100 mg DMAE
100 mcg chromium picolinate
60 mg ginkgo biloba
1-5 mg thiamin (vitamin B_1)
1-9 mg riboflavin (vitamin B_2)
20 mg vitamin B_3 (niacinamide)
100 mg vitamin B_5 (pantothenic acid)
2 mg vitamin B_6 (pyridoxine)
1,000 mcg vitamin B_{12}

1,000 mg vitamin C
400 mcg folic acid
15 mg coenzyme Q_{10}
100 mg caffeine (use green tea extract when possible)
8 oz serving of any sweet beverage of your choice, such as fruit juice, or a beverage sweetened with NutraSweet.
400 IU vitamin E

1. Crush all tablets (you may also take capsules or tablets separately if desired) until they are the consistency of fine powder (use a food processor or a mortar and pestle, if available).
2. Put the powder in a blender with 2–4 ice cubes and pour in cold juice or a pre-sweetened beverage.
3. Blend until smooth.

1 SERVING

When to Use the Choline Cocktail

I use this smart cocktail each day before interviews, personal appearances, debates, and lectures; while I write; and before I read scientific journals. I find that within thirty minutes to an hour of drinking it, I am more focused and energized and can more easily assimilate and recall facts.

I suggest that you try it as a morning beverage in place of coffee. Use it again after lunch to avoid midday mental fatigue. Choline should be avoided by people with psychotic disorders, such as manic-depressive psychosis, those with type A (high-strung or aggressive) personalities, and those on medications that affect the cholinergic nervous system. Persons with the inherited metabolic disorder PKU (phenylketonuria) should not use NutraSweet or Equal or nutritional supplements that contain L-phenylalanine.

How to Boost Acetylcholine in the Brain with Foods

People who want to use ordinary foods instead of dietary supplements to increase levels of the energy and memory neurotransmitters acetylcholine and norepinephrine in the brain should choose from the following lists of selected smart foods that are rich in the nutrients required for synthesizing acetylcholine. These foods supply choline, vitamin C, and vitamin B_5 (along with smaller amounts of vitamin B_6 and zinc) that can help optimize the conversion of dietary choline into acetylcholine in the brain. You can increase the release of norepinephrine in the brain by consuming one to two cups of green tea or coffee in conjunction with the smart foods listed next.

Choline-rich Foods

Choline doesn't have to compete with other nutrients, such as amino acids, to enter the brain. Most healthy people in the United States consume 600 to 1,000 milligrams per day of choline (as free choline and lecithin). Make your selections, as desired, from the following list of smart foods:

Choline-rich Foods (in mg)

Wheat germ (½ cup)	2,820
Peanuts (½ cup)	1,113
Peanut butter (½ cup)	966
Calf's liver (3.5 ounces)	850
Ham (3.5 ounces)	800
Lamb chops (3.5 ounces)	753
Whole wheat flour (½ cup)	613
White rice (½ cup)	586
Trout (3.5 ounces)	580
Beef (eye round) (3.5 ounces)	453
Whole egg (1 large)	394
White flour (½ cup)	346
Pecans (½ cup)	333

Vitamin C–rich Foods

Vitamin C plays an essential role in mind fitness. Your brain requires extraordinarily large amounts of vitamin C to operate at optimal levels for two reasons. First, it needs vitamin C (a potent water-soluble antioxidant that works synergistically with the fat-soluble antioxidant vitamin E) to prevent free-radical damage from the high concentration of unsaturated fats in brain cells (these unsaturated fats are especially susceptible to oxidation). Second, it requires vitamin C for the synthesis of neuro-transmitters, such as norepinephrine, dopamine, and acetylcholine. Vita-min C is so important to healthy brain function that the brain has evolved specialized vitamin C "pumps" that concentrate the vitamin at ten to fifteen times the levels found in the blood.

Some nutritionists point out that the most efficient and economical way to take vitamin C supplements and achieve maximum absorption is to ingest three equally divided doses of 1 gram (3 grams per day). For example, if you take 1 gram of vitamin C in a single dose, you will absorb 75 percent of the dose. With a dose of 2 grams, your body will absorb only 44 percent; 3 grams, 39 percent; 4 grams, 28 percent; and 5 grams, 20 percent. Therefore, by taking 1 gram of vitamin C three times each day, you will absorb enough of the vitamin to achieve maximum mental performance (about 2 grams per day). (I don't recommend time-release vitamin C or any other time-release supplement because of inconsistent degradation in the gastrointestinal tract.) You may also be able to lower your blood cholesterol level (vitamin C helps break down cholesterol and convert it to bile acids), fight stress (your adrenal glands, which produce hormones under stressful conditions, use up large amounts of vitamin C to do so), and protect your arteries against free-radical damage (vitamin C is a potent antioxidant that promotes cardiovascular health. In addition, large doses of vitamin C have been shown, in the laboratory, to prevent many types of environmentally caused cancers.

I have met hundreds of physicians and dietitians around the world who privately consume megadoses of vitamin C, but publicly caution against taking nutritional supplements ("You can get all the vitamin C you need from foods," they claim). They're afraid of professional ostracism and ridicule because the professional organizations to which they belong still hold that nutritional supplements are unnecessary and are just another health-food fad. Although a number of Nobel laureates, physicians, dieti-tians, and distinguished scientists the world over now believe that this orthodox view should be changed, fear of political "incorrectness" still intimidates many of them, so they continue to repeat the "party line" of most national health organizations.

I take several grams of vitamin C each day because it is probably the single-most-important nutrient that can help reduce the risk of many degenerative diseases and improve the mental and physical quality of life. A wealth of published research supports my view. Anyone who claims that this amount of vitamin C is "wasted" is, in my opinion, out of touch with the reality of contemporary scientific evidence.

I don't want to give the impression, however, that you should simply take vitamin C supplements and disregard eating vitamin C–rich foods. These foods contain many other valuable nutrients, such as polyphenols or bioflavonoids and fiber. That's why you should include the following vitamin C–rich foods in your regular diet:

Vitamin C Content of Selected Foods (in mg)

Broccoli (1 cup, steamed)	70–160
Brussels sprouts (1 cup, steamed)	90–150
Cauliflower (1 cup, raw)	50–90
Strawberries (1 cup)	40–90
Lemons (1 large)	50–80
Cabbage (1 cup, raw)	50–80
Oranges (1 medium)	40–60
Grapefruit ($\frac{1}{2}$ medium)	35–45
Pineapples (1 cup)	20–40
Turnips (1 cup, cooked)	15–40
Tomatoes (1 raw)	10–30
Peaches (1 medium)	5–25
Potatoes (1 medium, cooked)	10–20
Beans ($\frac{1}{2}$ cup, cooked)	10–20
Peas ($\frac{1}{2}$ cup, cooked)	10–15
Apples (1 medium)	5–10
Bananas (1 medium)	5–10

Pantothenic Acid–rich Foods

Pantothenic acid, also known as vitamin B_5, is ubiquitous in nature because it is synthesized by most microorganisms and plants. It is particularly abundant in meat, fish, poultry, beans, peas, lentils, and whole-grain cereals. Two cholesterol-rich foods, egg yolks and liver, contain large amounts of pantothenic acid. Healthier foods sources include broccoli, skim milk, and sweet potatoes.

Pantothenic acid is an important part of the molecule acetyl-coenzyme A, which plays a central role in the brain's energy production. As I mentioned earlier, pantothenic acid is also required for the synthesis of the brain neurotransmitter acetylcholine, an important mind-fitness nutrient associated with mental energy and memory enhancement. Research studies reveal that pantothenic acid also helps the body handle stress. American adults, on the average, get about 7 milligrams per day from ordinary foods. Some scientists believe that maximum mental performance requires much higher intakes, in the range of 200 to 500 milligrams per day. Use the following foods to increase your intake of this mind-fitness nutrient:

Pantothenic Acid (Vitamin B₅) Content of Selected Foods (in mg)

Egg yolk (1 medium)	100–200
Kidney (3.5 ounces)	100–200
Liver (3.5 ounces)	100–200
Yeast (½ cup)	100–200
Broccoli (1 cup, cooked)	35–100
Beef (3.5 ounces)	35–100
Skim milk (1 cup)	35–100
Sweet potato (1 medium)	35–100
Molasses (½ cup)	35–100

3

Effortless Weight Loss:

The Eat Smart, Think Smart 🔥 *Meltdown Formula*

What's a chapter on weight loss doing in a book about smart nutrients?

By now, you've seen what a profound connection there is between the mind and the body. The fact is, body metabolism and muscle function are affected as much by smart nutrients as are mental alertness, creativity, and memory. Harnessing the full power of smart nutrients means enjoying an amazing range of physical, as well as mental and emotional, benefits.

This combination of smart nutrients can help you to lose fat and maintain muscle *without changing your current diet.* In other words, keep eating as you're eating now, but take the Meltdown Formula, and you will still lose weight.

More than likely, you've found yourself longing for a little less body fat. Like many people, you may be caught in a vicious cycle of gaining and losing weight. Even if you've failed repeatedly to keep lost weight off, the fat-burning smart-nutrient formula I'm going to tell you about will help you reach your target weight and stay there.

But first, let's learn exactly how smart nutrients work to achieve weight loss. Then you'll learn how to create the Meltdown Formula from supplements you can get in any health food store, vitamin shop, or pharmacy—or you can purchase premixed meltdown-type formulas from sources listed in

Appendix I. Next, you'll learn about some additional vitamin and mineral supplements that more and more research is finding play an important role not only in weight loss and maintenance but in overall health. Finally, you'll get a set of guidelines for the kinds of foods you should be eating to create the best, healthiest base for achieving and sustaining your ideal weight.

Rev Up Your Fat Furnace

My revolutionary fat-burning smart-nutrient mix, the Meltdown Formula, uses a unique combination of thermogenic (fat-burning) and muscle-building (anabolic) smart nutrients that work together to get you thin and keep you thin.

I know, I know. Many of you have regained all the weight you've lost on past diets and weight-loss schemes. It's hard to live forever on yogurt and alfalfa sprouts. To all of you who enjoy a variety of foods and cuisines, from the ordinary to the sublime, take heart. The Meltdown Formula is the smart fat-burning strategy to use, especially if you enjoy your present way of eating. It works with your regular diet, as long as your weight has stabilized. For example, if you are 25 pounds overweight and have been at that weight for at least two to three months, your body will begin mobilizing fat within twenty minutes of starting the plan and will continue to burn fat for as long as you follow the plan. Regular exercise (which I highly recommend) is not required for fat loss on this plan; however, the muscle-building (anabolic) effects of the plan can be achieved only with exercise.

The formula also elevates your mood and stimulates the brain and nervous system to reach maximum mental performance while you burn fat. Remember, *you won't have to change the way you like to eat for this formula to work*. Of course, the healthy way of eating I recommend in all my books (a low-fat, low-cholesterol, moderate-protein, high-carbohydrate diet and regular exercise) can help you achieve your weight-loss and health goals even faster.

The Fat-burning Formula with Muscle

The Meltdown Formula uses your body's natural thermogenic and an-abolic mechanisms to achieve two essential goals: fat burning and muscle maintenance or growth (depending upon whether you exercise). Here's how it works:

THERMOGENIC SMART NUTRIENTS. Each cell in your body contains a furnace (called a mitochondrion) for burning fat. Fuel the furnace with the proper combination of thermogenic smart nutrients, and it will burn extra body fat (biochemists call this process "uncoupling oxidation from phosphorylation"; you'll call it a miracle). Thermogenesis is actually the process by which your body generates heat from fat.

That brings me to an important point: Anything that generates body heat—spices, hot foods, a sauna bath, exercise, and thermogenic smart nutrients—will cause your body to burn fat. Every time you raise your body's internal temperature, you tell it to burn fat. A fundamental principle of biochemistry is that *whatever heats you up, slims you down.* By regularly using thermogenic smart nutrients, your body revs up its fat-burning furnace. Fat loss is not as much a matter of special diet as it is of causing your body to enter a fat-burning state. The Meltdown Formula will help you do just that.

ANABOLIC SMART NUTRIENTS. The search for safe and natural alternatives to steroid drugs among professional athletes has led to the discovery of anabolic (muscle-building) smart nutrients. Although anabolic smart nutrients won't build additional muscle unless you exercise, even basic movements, such as walking and lifting, can help confirmed couch potatoes maintain at least some of their muscle as they lose fat with anabolic smart nutrients. Since muscle is the primary metabolic tissue that burns fat, it makes sense to maintain as much of it as possible. *Weight loss without muscle growth or maintenance is a major reason why many people regain lost weight.*

Most weight-loss programs cause you to lose a significant amount of muscle along with fat. On ordinary weight-loss diets, you often reach your target weight at the expense of muscle loss, which also means a loss in your body's ability to burn fat at the rate you enjoyed when you started your diet. The Meltdown Formula contains anabolic smart nutrients that burn fat and maintain or increase (depending upon your level of exercise) your ratio of muscle to fat. When you reach your ideal body weight, you'll have more muscle to help you keep the weight from returning.

Tennis Anyone?

Ivan Lendl, world-champion tennis star, was amazed. Even his athletically toned body could not stop the power of fat-burning smart nutrients. Each day for one month, Ivan ate a smart-nutrient "snack" containing thermogenic and anabolic smart nutrients. In just four weeks, he lost ten pounds without changing the way he ate. Ivan's smart-nutrient snack included chromium picolinate (a patented mineral formulation designed by a scientist at the U.S. Department of Agriculture), which helped him gain several pounds of muscle tissue (because of his strength-training regimen).

Ivan's experience with thermogenic and anabolic smart nutrients is similar to Cher's and Glenn Frey's (of the legendary rock group The Eagles). For example, when I first began working with Cher, who had gained twenty pounds after a demanding movie role, I gave her a prototype of the Meltdown Formula. "You can be my first real-world guinea pig," I told her. She was so thrilled with the results that she forgave my poor choice of words—I think.

Everyone I've worked with has used smart nutrients to achieve personal weight-loss goals (for even greater benefit, they also rely on exercise to improve their muscle strength, tone, and overall health). In the following section, I'll show you how to create your own Meltdown Formula to help you achieve the success enjoyed by my clients. You may not aspire to win the U.S. Open tennis championship or want to win an Oscar, but there's nothing wrong with looking and feeling as if you could!

Before You Begin the Meltdown Formula

Excess body fat is associated with an elevated risk of certain types of cancer, cardiovascular disease, gallstones, diabetes, and hypertension, so it makes good sense to take off extra pounds and keep them off, but not at the expense of yo-yo dieting—continually losing and gaining weight in a vicious cycle of success and failure. This formula will give you a fighting chance to lose weight and keep it off. It can be used to lose up to 25 pounds by following these guidelines:

1. *Check with your physician before using the formula* to determine if there is any medical reason (such as high blood pressure, cardiovascular disease, prostate problems, peptic ulcer disease, or bleeding disorders) why you should not take the formula.
2. Use the recommended vitamin-mineral once-a-day supplement formula to maximize fat loss (detailed later in this chapter).
3. The Meltdown Formula is not a license to overeat or to base your diet on junk food. Follow a sensible and nutritious low-fat eating plan, with plenty of whole grains, fresh fruits, and vegetables (see my books *Eat to Win* and *Eat to Succeed* for the complete plans I recommend) for best results.

4. Any weight-loss–weight-maintenance plan works best with regular exercise—even a thirty to sixty-minute walk each day can work wonders for your health and waistline. The lack of exercise, however, will not block the fat-burning effects of the formula.

Since everyone is biochemically unique, the weight loss results will vary. Published studies that have examined thermogenesis-induced weight loss reveal impressive results when thermogenic compounds, such as caffeine and ephedra, are combined with a low-calorie diet (for example, 1,000 kilocalories per day).

The Meltdown Formula

You can purchase the ingredients to make your own Meltdown-type formula at most health food stores and pharmacies; you can also purchase it premixed, as a smart drink, from various manufacturers (see Appendix I for the manufacturers' names, addresses, and telephone numbers).

The most convenient way to use the Meltdown Formula is to combine three products (available in most health food stores and vitamin shops):

Twin Lab's Choline Cocktail (Twin Laboratories) powdered beverage mix

Trim-Time Thermogenic Tea (Alvita brand) or any thermogenic ephedra tea made by a variety of manufacturers; see Appendix I.

Combine one tablespoon each of QuickFix and Twin Lab's Choline Cocktail in one cup of ephedra tea. Ordinary choline supplements taste and smell awful, but Twin Lab's Choline Cocktail contains a flavor system that renders it tasteless and odorless.

If you decide to make the formula from scratch, follow the recipe in the next section.

A Recipe for Successful Fat Loss

If you decide to make your own version of the Meltdown Formula, follow this daily plan for optimal fat loss:

BREAKFAST. Drink one cup of thermogenic ephedra tea in the morning with a low-fat breakfast, such as whole-grain cereal, skim milk, and fresh fruit.

Take the following ingredients with breakfast:

- L-carnitine capsule (250 mg)
- Chromium picolinate capsule (200 mcg)
- Potassium-magnesium phosphate: one glass of Endurance brand QuickFix (available at health food stores and vitamin shops) or take a 1g potassium-magnesium phosphate capsule supplement (see Appendix I for suppliers)

LUNCH. Drink another cup of ephedra tea with a low-fat protein meal, such as a turkey sandwich on whole-grain bread with lettuce, tomato, and mustard plus one serving of fresh fruit. Take all additional supplements (L-carnitine, chromium picolinate, and potassium phosphate) as described, again with lunch.

Thermogenic Green Tea Promotes Fat Loss and Health

With the exception of water, green tea is the most commonly consumed beverage in the world (although it is not widely consumed by people in the United States). Trim-Time Thermogenic Tea contains five fat-burning thermogenic substances: ephedrine, salicin, caffeine, ginger, and cayenne pepper. The health-giving benefits of green tea, however, derive from the polyphenols it contains. Polyphenols are antioxidant compounds that have been shown to protect laboratory animals from a variety of diseases and environmental toxins.

The following is a list of the known benefits of polyphenols derived from green tea and green tea extracts (available in capsules from most health foods stores and mail-order companies: see Appendix I).

Green tea polyphenols can:

- help stimulate the process of thermogenesis to aid in body-fat loss
- afford many times the antioxidant activity of vitamin E in preventing free-radical damage to the brain
- work synergistically with vitamins C and E to provide greater antioxidant protection
- provide a 45 percent reduction in the risk of lung cancer for cigarette smokers
- protect against UV light–induced skin damage
- inhibit platelet activity factor (PAF), which causes platelet clumping

that can initiate a heart attack or stroke (this inhibition is similar to that afforded by the smart herb, ginkgo biloba).
- lower LDL cholesterol and elevate HDL cholesterol
- lower blood pressure through inhibition of the angiotensin-converting enzyme
- reduce the risk of bacterial food poisoning, dental caries, and gingivitis
- block blood-sugar elevation by inhibiting the enzyme, amylase which the body uses to absorb sugar from starch
- inhibit the growth of the influenza virus. Research is currently being conducted using green-tea extracts to inhibit the replication of the AIDS virus.

Trim-Time Thermogenic Tea (Alvita brand) contains willow bark (salacin), an ingredient similar to ordinary aspirin. Published studies have shown that aspirin aids the thermogenic process and speeds up body-fat loss when used in conjunction with ephedra and caffeine, but the Meltdown Formula will work fine without it. Certain individuals may be aspirin sensitive or may have medical conditions (or be taking medications) for which aspirin is contraindicated. *Check with a physician before taking aspirin or any other ingredient in the Meltdown Formula.*

EPHEDRA. Ephedra is a naturally occurring herbal compound used in the Orient for thousands of years. It is available in the United States as an over-the-counter smart-nutrient supplement, most often found in teas and herbal products. Ephedra contains ephedrine, an ingredient found in over-the-counter cold decongestants. Studies that have examined the thermogenic effects of ephedra and ephedrine have revealed that they can, indeed, accelerate the burning of fat. Olympic athletes are prohibited from using ephedra- or ephedrine-containing compounds, such as asthma medications, because these substances can give them an unfair advantage in their performance. Any athlete who is found using ephedra or ephedrine is automatically disqualified from competition. Professional bodybuilders, however, can and do use ma huang (an ephedrine-containing herb) to "get ripped"—bodyspeak for burning fat to reveal underlying muscle tone.

Dosage commonly used: one to two cups of ephedra tea per day.

Do not use ephedra or products that contain ephedrine, such as thermogenic tea, if you are pregnant, lactating, have high blood pressure, cardiovascular disease including cardiac arrhythmia, diabetes, glaucoma, prostatitic hypertrophy, hyperthyroidism or other thyroid condition, or psychosis. Elderly persons may be extrasensitive to tea containing ma huang. People taking prescription medications such as anorectics, MAO inhibitor drugs, other antidepressants, or cardiovascular medications should consult a physician before using ma huang or products that contain it.

L-CARNITINE. Without this smart nutrient, your body can't burn even an ounce of fat. L-carnitine actually transports fat into the fat-burning furnace in each cell. Although your body can manufacture a certain amount of L-carnitine each day, research has shown that certain conditions, such as aging, high-fat or high-protein consumption, exercise, stress, steroid use, illness, alcohol ingestion, and the synthesis of glycogen (the storage form of carbohydrate), may deplete your body's supply of it. One recent study also demonstrated that L-carnitine may act as an ergogenic (energy-giving) substance that improves endurance in trained athletes, most likely by stimulating the synthesis of the energy molecule, ATP.

Dosage commonly used: 250–500 mg per day.

METHYL XANTHINES (GREEN TEA, COFFEE). Green tea (found in health food stores and oriental groceries) contains caffeine and related methyl xanthine compounds that can increase the body's metabolic rate. Caffeine can also stimulate the release of stored body fat, allowing it, instead of carbohydrates, to be burned. Methyl xanthines in green tea and coffee increase thermogenesis, causing the body to burn fat, rather than carbohydrates, for fuel. Published studies have shown that most healthy people can safely consume up to 200 milligrams of caffeine per day.

Dosage commonly used: Up to 200 mg per day (about two cups of green tea or brewed coffee).

POTASSIUM, MAGNESIUM, AND PHOSPHATE. Scientists recently discovered a relationship between fat burning and three common nutrients: phosphates and the minerals potassium and magnesium. In one study, women who drank orange juice enriched with potassium, magnesium, and phosphate increased their metabolic rate and experienced high rates of thermogenesis after meals (called postprandial thermogenesis).

I've been using potassium- and magnesium phosphate for almost a decade to help professional athletes burn excess body fat and improve their physical endurance and performance. Martina Navratilova used this mixture to win her Wimbledon championships, and Ivan Lendl used it when he won his U.S. Open title. Cher and other motion-picture celebrities have also used this smart nutrient to rev up and slim down.

The popular press has just "discovered" the energy and weight-loss benefits of potassium- and magnesium phosphates, but these benefits should come as no surprise to my loyal readers (I revealed the high-energy benefits of their use almost a decade ago in my book *Eat to Succeed*). Although the long-term efficacy of these minerals remains to be proved in scientific studies, I have seen the results firsthand in my clients since I began recommending these nutrients. Potassium- and magnesium phosphate supplements are sold in health food stores throughout the United States.

Dosage commonly used: 500–2,000 mg per day.

CHROMIUM PICOLINATE. Chromium picolinate, developed by a scientist at the U.S. Department of Agriculture, is a trace-element compound that helps regulate blood-sugar levels. The body absorbs this special form of the mineral chromium several times better than it does inorganic chromium salts. One study demonstrated that 200 micrograms of chromium picolinate per day increased lean body mass (muscle) in female college students who participated in a supervised weight-reduction program. Because of their larger body weight and lean muscle mass, men may require slightly more chromium picolinate to achieve a similar effect. Used in conjunction with the Meltdown Formula, chromium picolinate can help minimize the corresponding muscle loss that usually accompanies weight loss. Just as important, it can help build muscle tissue (with exercise) during periods of reduced calorie intake.

Dosage commonly used: 200–400 mcg per day.

As was mentioned earlier, aspirin, by itself, can help stoke each cell's fat-burning furnace; research has shown that a low dose of aspirin (about one tablet, or 325 milligrams) can speed the loss of body fat by promoting thermogenesis. If you use aspirin with ephedra and caffeine, two other thermogenic smart substances you've already learned about, the fat-burning process accelerates even more.

> Aspirin is not an essential ingredient of the Meltdown Formula, but if both are used concurrently, with your physician's permission, they can hasten the fat-burning process.
>
> *Dosage commonly used:* one to two tablets (325–650 mg per day).

> **CAUTION:** The Meltdown Formula contains ingredients that may be contraindicated in certain individuals. Although people have used caffeine and ephedra for thousands of years, some individuals may be sensitive to these or other ingredients in the formula. Always check with your physician before beginning this or any other dietary program. Do not take this warning lightly. An ounce of prevention is worth a pound of cure—or body fat, for that matter!

Ancillary Smart Nutrients for Healthy Weight Loss

Reduced-calorie diets and thermogenic substances can increase your body's need for a variety of nutrients, especially those involved with fat burning, energy production, and protecting cells against free-radical damage. To date, no one has devised a method for determining your body's unique need for all known nutrients, a need that fluctuates according to your age, sex, level of physical activity, illness, previous diet, and many other parameters. Nutritional supplementation is still a hotly debated issue among nutritionists. I believe that supplementation with a multivitamin–mineral formula can help make up for any nutritional deficiencies in your diet, as well as help protect against a host of health problems, including cardiovascular disease, certain types of cancer, and premature aging of the brain.

Here is a list of nutrients, including vitamins, minerals, and non-vitamin nutrients (such as coenzyme Q_{10}, choline, inositol, and biotin) that I believe promote optimal health. In general, people who are following a reduced-calorie regimen, that is, are attempting to lose weight, should find a nutritional supplement that contains the nutrients listed in Chart 3.1.

CHART 3.1
Recommended Nutritional Supplement Formula
(see Appendix I for information on manufacturers)

Look for a daily vitamin-mineral supplement that contains the following ingredients in these approximate dosages:

Coenzyme Q_{10} (30 mg)
Vitamin A acetate (5,000 IU)
Vitamin D_3 (200 IU)
Beta-carotene (25,000 IU)
Vitamin E (400 IU)
Vitamin C (1,000 mg)
Ascorbyl palmitate (100 mg)
Bioflavonoid complex
Vitamin B_1 (25 mg)
Vitamin B_2 (25 mg)
Vitamin B_6 (75 mg)
Vitamin B_3 (125 mg)
Pantothenic acid (100 mg)
Vitamin B_{12} (100 mcg)
Folic acid (800 mcg)

Biotin (300 mcg)
PABA (10 mg)
Choline bitartrate (225 mg)
Inositol (100 mg)
Calcium (800 mg)*
Magnesium (400 mg)
Zinc (30 mg)
Manganese (10 mg)
Copper (2 mg)
Selenium (200 mcg)
Chromium picolinate (200 mcg)
Molybdenum (250 mcg)
L-cysteine (250 mg)
L-methionine (100 mg)
L-glutathione (50 mg)

* May require additional supplementation to get this amount.

Persons with Wilson's disease (an inherited condition characterized by excessive copper storage) should not take any nutritional supplement containing copper without first checking with a physician.

Anyone taking large doses of vitamin E should consult an ophthalmologist to make sure they don't have retinitis pigmentosa (half of those who develop RP have no idea that they're at risk because it's a recessive trait). More information on RP can be obtained from the RP Foundation (800-683-5555). Persons who take vitamin E supplements should inform their physicians before any scheduled surgery because vitamin E can prolong bleeding times.

You can reach your target weight using the Meltdown Formula without changing the way you eat, but let's face it, thinness is not synonymous with health. I want you to lose excess body fat, but not at the expense of good health. The primary purposes of fat loss, after all, are to look good, feel good about yourself, and reduce your risk of diseases, such as cancer, heart problems, hypertension, and diabetes.

In the mid-1970s, I began an ambitious quest to change the eating habits of this country. When I first tried to tell leading health authorities that too much fat, cholesterol, and protein were the primary culprits in the American diet, few took me seriously. Today, nearly fifteen years later, dietitians, physicians, and other health-care professionals now recommend that everyone follow the type of dietary principles I espoused in *Eat to Win*. These principles can give you the healthy nutrition your body requires during weight loss and weight maintenance.

The smart-food exchange lists that follow will help you enjoy low-fat, low-cholesterol eating along with the Meltdown Formula. Enjoy these foods as desired (and the smart recipes in Chapter 9) to help you reach your target weight safely and effectively.

Eat to Lose: Burning Fat with Protein and Carbohydrates

Smart foods are rich in complex carbohydrates and high-quality protein, but poor in fat—a winning combination for good health, fat loss, and maximum mental performance. These are the foods that contribute to a lifetime of health, mental and physical fitness, and youthful vitality.

I've created the following easy-to-follow exchange lists to help you choose the healthiest foods that contain a rich supply of smart nutrients. Use them whenever possible to achieve maximal weight loss; use them just as liberally to help maintain your target weight and optimal health.

Eat Smart, Think Smart Food-Exchange Lists

PROTEIN (FOUR EXCHANGES PER DAY). High-quality protein foods contain a rich supply of the amino acids (including L-phenylalanine and L-tyrosine) that the brain requires to manufacture vital neurotransmitters, such as norepinephrine and dopamine. You can enjoy an abundant supply of these and other important amino acids by combining the recommended animal and vegetable protein sources.

Each protein-food portion listed below contains one exchange within its group (four exchanges are recommended each day):

Meat Exchanges (four per day)

- Beef (round steak or flank steak—"select grade," lowest in fat) with visible fat trimmed: 1 ounce
- Fish: 1 ounce or ¼ cup canned albacore tuna, packed in water
- Chicken (without skin): 1 ounce
- Turkey (without skin): 1 ounce
- Pork tenderloin (all visible fat trimmed): 1 ounce

When selecting foods from the protein-exchange category, keep in mind the following order of desirability:

Fish and shellfish (except shrimp) come first because they are the lowest in fat and contain no more cholesterol than beef, pork, and other high-protein foods. For example, a 4-ounce serving of steamed lobster contains about 90 milligrams of cholesterol and 2 grams of fat; by comparison, a 4-ounce serving of lean beef contains about 100 milligrams of cholesterol and 8 grams of fat. Shrimp, naturally low in fat, contains about 130 milligrams of cholesterol per 4-ounce serving, so it should be eaten in no more than a 3-ounce portion.

Chicken or turkey (white meat without skin) is your next choice because it is relatively low in fat, although it contains as much cholesterol per serving as do most servings of fish and beef (about 27 milligrams of cholesterol per ounce).

Beef and pork are last on the animal-protein list because of their higher total fat content, especially saturated fat, which tends to raise blood cholesterol levels. You can keep the fat content down, however, by purchasing "select-grade" meats, instead of "prime"- or "choice"-grade meats when possible. Round steak and flank steak, in any grade, are generally the lowest in fat.

Nonfat or Low-Fat (1 or 2 percent) Dairy Exchanges (two per day)

- Yogurt: 6 ounces
- Dry-curd cottage cheese: 2 ounces
- Hoop cheese: 2 ounces
- Milk: 8 ounces
- Nonfat buttermilk: 8 ounces
- Evaporated milk: 4 ounces
- Powdered milk: ⅓ cup

Two nonfat or low-fat dairy servings each day are recommended because these foods are an excellent source of calcium, protein, and vitamins A, D, and B_{12}. Each nonfat or low-fat milk product in this exchange group contains about 90 calories.

Even though we need to eat protein each day, too much protein can adversely affect kidney and liver function, may cause kidney stones, can raise blood cholesterol levels, and may be associated with an increased risk of certain types of diet-related cancer. Bear in mind that almost everything we eat contains protein, so the daily protein allowance of about 45 grams for women and 55 grams for men (although recent research suggests that some bodybuilders may require an additional 10 to 20 grams per day) can easily be met by eating a varied diet that contains grains, cereals, vegetables, nonfat milk products, and small portions (100 grams or 3½ ounces) of chicken, turkey, seafood, or lean beef or pork.

Lacto-ovo vegetarians, who consume nonfat milk products and eggs (preferably only egg whites) can easily meet their daily protein needs by eating these foods in addition to a variety of vegetables, grains, fruits, and potatoes or other starchy tubers. Studies have shown that, in general, vegetarians enjoy lower rates of heart disease, cancer, diabetes, kidney stones, kidney and liver diseases, and obesity than do omnivores. If you are a lacto-ovo vegetarian, you can easily follow the Eat Smart, Think Smart exchange system and still be assured that you are embracing a nutritionally balanced eating plan.

For vegetarians and those who follow a low-fat–low-cholesterol diet, the following high-protein foods contain no cholesterol and little fat:

Beans, peas, and lentils (these foods are included under the complex-carbohydrate exchange list as well because they provide a rich source of both complex carbohydrate and protein: ½ cup equals one protein exchange).

Egg whites (about four per day, two egg whites = one protein exchange).

CARBOHYDRATE EXCHANGES. This is the most liberal of the exchange groups because these are the foods that supply the most nutrition for the least calories. Complex carbohydrate foods (as opposed to simple carbohydrate foods (sugars and sweeteners) contain dietary fiber, which is essential to your health. Dietary fiber can help reduce blood cholesterol levels and lower the risk of diet-related cancer and adult-onset diabetes. Fiber also adds bulk to the diet, which aids in regularity and imparts a sense of fullness after a meal.

Unlike protein and fat, complex carbohydrates burn cleanly, leaving behind no toxic metabolic waste products as do protein and fat. Increasing the amount of complex carbohydrates in the diet automatically reduces the amount of fat, thereby helping to reduce one's tendency to gain weight, and helps lower the risk of cardiovascular disease, cancer, diabetes, and a host of degenerative diseases.

Complex Carbohydrate Exchanges (four per day)

- Breads: 1 slice, or 1 ounce
- Grains, cooked: ½ cup
- Cereal: ⅓ to ½ cup
- Pastas: ½ cup
- Beans, peas, lentils: ½ cup

Here are some examples of common complex-carbohydrate foods:

Rice (preferably brown) and all other whole grains
Whole-grain breakfast cereals made without fat
Pasta (made without egg yolks): all types, including spaghetti, linguini, macaroni, and lasagna noodles
Beans—all types (soybeans should be limited because of their high fat content)
Peas—all types (chick-peas should be limited because of their high fat content)
Lentils (all types)
Potatoes (white and sweet)
Yams
Corn
All whole-grain baking flours
Cornstarch and arrowroot

GREEN AND YELLOW VEGETABLE EXCHANGES (UP TO FOUR PER DAY). On the Eat Smart, Think Smart exchange plan, vegetables play an important role because they contain the most smart nutrients for the fewest calories of all foods.

Some vegetables, such as spinach, are richly endowed with nearly the same amino-acid profile (a measure of protein quality) as is beef (see Chart 3.2). So don't be misled into thinking that vegetables contain "inferior" protein. Consider this: The steak that you enjoyed last night for dinner

CHART 3.2
Essential Amino-Acid Profile of Spinach and Steak

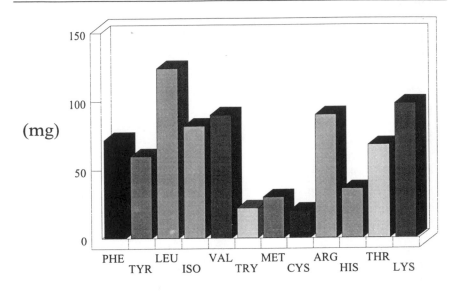

Spinach, Raw (1 cup)

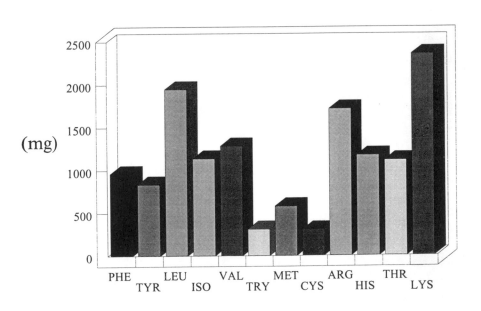

Sirloin Steak, Broiled (3.5 ounces)

PHE=phenylalanine, LEU=leucine, VAL=valine, MET=methionine, ARG=arginine, THR=threonine, TYR=tyrosine, ISO=isoleucine, TRY=tryptophan, CYS-cysteine, HIS=histidine, and LYS= lysine.

came from a steer that never ate meat. And don't forget that many vegetarian world-champion athletes have built award-winning muscles from eating vegetables.

Vegetables also contain fiber, vitamins, minerals, and compounds that help reduce the risk of diet-related cancer. Beta-carotene, for example, is the form of vitamin A found in the vegetable kingdom. Research has suggested that it and other substances found in cruciferous vegetables (such as cauliflower and cabbage) can go a long way toward preventing and even reversing some of the early changes in the body that can lead to cancer.

The following vegetables can be eaten in portions of ½ cup: artichoke, asparagus, bean sprouts, beets, beet greens, bok choy, broccoli, brussels sprouts, cabbage, carrots, cauliflower, celery, chard, chicory, collard greens, cucumbers, dandelion greens, eggplant, endive, escarole, green pepper, Jerusalem artichoke, kale, leeks, lettuce (all types), mustard greens, okra, onions, parsley, pea pods (Chinese), pumpkin, radishes, rhubarb, rutabaga, spaghetti squash, spinach, summer squash, tomatoes, turnips, turnip greens, watercress, winter squash, and zucchini.

FRUIT EXCHANGES (UP TO FOUR PER DAY). Fruits, like vegetables, are good sources of fiber, and they're low in fat. They contain no cholesterol, and because of their high water content, are low in calories.

Since many fresh fruits contain appreciable amounts of natural sugar (simple carbohydrates), you should limit your intake to four exchanges per day. Very active people can add additional fruit—up to two or more additional exchanges each day. Frozen or canned fruits, packed without sugar or syrup, are also recommended. Note that dried fruits are more concentrated sources of sugar, and so their exchange equivalent is half that of fresh fruit. Here is a list of fresh, frozen, and unsweetened canned fruit and fruit-juice exchanges:

Fruits: apple (fresh: 1 small, about 2½-inch diameter; dried, 4 rings), applesauce (unsweetened: ½ cup), apricots (fresh: 4 medium; dried: 6 halves), banana (½ medium), berries (blueberries, raspberries, and so on: ¾ cup), cantaloupe (5-inch diameter, ⅓ melon), cherries (large, 12), cherries (canned, ½ cup), dates (2 medium), figs (fresh: 2, 2-inch diameter; dried: 2 small), fruit cocktail (canned: ½ cup), grapefruit (½ medium), grapes (15 small), honeydew melon (⅛) melon, cubed, 1 cup), kiwi (1 large), kumquats (5), mandarin oranges (¾ cup), mango (½ small), nectarine (1 medium, 1½-inch diameter), orange (1 medium, 2-inch diameter), papaya (1 cup), peach (1 medium, 2½-inch diameter, or ¾ cup), pear

(½ large or 1 small), pineapple (fresh: ¾ cup), plantain (½ small), plums (2, 2-inch diameter), prunes (fresh: 2 medium; dried: 3), raisins (2 table-spoons), strawberries (fresh, 1¼ cups), tangerine (2, 2½-inch diameter), watermelon (1¼ cups cubed).

Fruit juices: apple juice or cider (½ cup), cranberry juice cocktail (⅓ cup), grapefruit juice (½ cup), grapefruit juice cocktail (⅓ cup), grape juice (½ cup), orange juice (½ cup), pineapple juice (½ cup), prune juice (⅓ cup).

The complex-carbohydrate exchange list is extensive and varied enough to afford anyone a nutritious and delicious way of achieving and maintaining optimal health and fitness. Complex carbohydrate foods—cereals, grains, vegetables, and fruits—can help you build a better, fitter, and healthier body. By applying the exchange principles outlined here, you can begin to establish lifelong eating patterns that help you achieve optimal health and maximum mental performance.

The following portions of complex-carbohydrate foods contain about 60 to 90 calories:

Breads

½ (average size) bagel (water, not egg)
1 slice bread (rye, whole-grain, French, white, sourdough)
1 hamburger bun
1 English muffin

Grains, Pastas, Cereals

½ cup barley (cooked)   ½ cup oatmeal (cooked)
½ cup whole-grain cereals   ½ cup rice (brown, cooked)
½ cup grits (cooked)   ½ cup spaghetti (cooked)
½ cup macaroni (cooked)

Vegetables

½ cup beans (cooked)   ½ cup peas (green, cooked)
½ cup corn (kernels, cooked)   1 cup potato (baked, average)
3 cups corn (hot-air popped)   ½ cup potato (mashed)
½ cup lentils (cooked)   ¾ cup squash (winter)

The complex-carbohydrate foods should make up from 60 percent to 80 percent of your total daily calories on the Eat Smart, Think Smart plan. These foods are relatively low in fat, sodium, and calories and contain no cholesterol. Complex carbohydrates are the only sources of fiber; vitamin E; and trace minerals, such as copper, manganese, and chromium—nutrients that research suggests can slow down the brain-aging process and help prevent degenerative diseases.

4

The Eat Smart, Think Smart Brain Antiaging Plan

The nutrient content of the ordinary diet won't defend your brain and other vital organs against the age-accelerating chemicals that lurk in our air, food, and water supply. You may eat a healthy diet and enjoy regular exercise to fight aging and fend off degenerative diseases, but without antioxidant smart nutrients, you're not protecting yourself from this environmental onslaught as effectively as possible.

I'm going to show you how to make the latest research on antioxidant smart nutrients work for you, first by focusing on what we now know about these antiaging nutrients, especially how they can prevent the damage that causes premature brain aging, with loss of memory and senility. Many of the mental disabilities that we attribute to ordinary aging can and should be prevented with antioxidant smart nutrients.

The antioxidant smart nutrient miniplan that I'll tell you about contains the very type of nutrients that can defend your brain and nervous system against chronic, lifelong free-radical damage. The pernicious nature of free-radical injury leads not only to brain dysfunction, but to other degenerative brain diseases, such as stroke and cancer. Antioxidant smart nutrients give you the chance to make a real difference in putting more life in your years and more years in your life. But first, what exactly are free radicals?

Free-Radical Pathology 101

Scientists have known for decades that free radicals (electrically charged atoms generated by every cell in the human body) attack the brain and central nervous system, damaging the delicate balance of chemistry and disrupting the fragile electronic network of nerves that allows us to think, feel, and act. Research over the past thirty years has implicated these atomic demons in a host of health problems, including memory loss, senility (including Alzheimer's disease), stroke, cancer, and massive nerve death that follows spinal-cord injury.

Free radicals are the price we pay for breathing, the inevitable consequence of living in a world where oxygen is the currency of nearly all life. Oxygen-related free radicals are a two-edged biological sword: We can't live with too many of them, and we can't live without enough of them. They are essential to a variety of metabolic reactions in the body involving the synthesis and metabolism of protein, fat, and carbohydrates. Our immune systems would be useless without the free radicals they generate to kill invading microbes. Left unchecked, however, free radicals can damage the delicate external framework of cells (called cell membranes or cell walls) and can cause cancer by injuring DNA, the genetic material that makes each of us unique.

A free radical is any atom that has an *unpaired* electron, an electrically charged particle that relentlessly searches for another electron "mate" to maintain stability and neutrality. When seemingly harmless substances, such as vegetable oil (or the highly unsaturated fats that make up brain cells), come in contact with free radicals, a chain reaction, or domino effect, may occur, creating thousands of additional free radicals that damage just about anything they touch. Free radicals cause fats to go rancid, turn bread into toast, turn a healthy brain into a senile one, and transform normal cells into cancerous ones.

Scientists first realized how free-radical damage could harm the brain by studying the hazards of radiation, particularly the type we receive from medical X-ray procedures. When X rays slam into the body, they split water molecules (most cells are about 90 percent water) into weak hydrogen-free radicals and extraordinarily destructive hydroxyl (one part oxygen and one part hydrogen) radicals. These hydroxyl radicals can destroy cell membranes in the brain and other organs, causing wholesale collapse of the cells; at the same time, they destroy the enzymes that repair DNA, which eventually leads to cancer.

In the late 1960s, scientists discovered one of the body's own defense systems against free radicals. This enzyme system, called SOD (superoxide dismutase), whose sole purpose is to neutralize a free radical called superoxide (a highly charged form of oxygen), plays an important role in the body's metabolism. It was then that scientists found that free radicals arise in the body not just under conditions of radioactive exposure, but during the daily processing of proteins, fats, and carbohydrates. In the mitochondria, the energy furnace of each cell, oxygen helps convert the digested foods we eat into usable fuel for the body, a process that ordinarily produces free radicals. Most of the free radicals are put to friendly metabolic purposes, such as building new biochemicals; others are neutralized by antioxidant systems, such as SOD. As it turns out, the mitochondrial membranes and their contents are especially susceptible to free-radical damage, and scientists now suspect that mitochondrial decay provides the origin of such age-related brain disorders as Parkinson's disease and senility.

Some white blood cells use free radicals to kill foreign microbes that invade the body. This type of free-radical production, however, is kept under tight control, eliminating the potential for cellular damage. A number of inflammatory conditions, including arthritis and severe infection, however, can cause white blood cells to gather and linger at the site of injury, leading to an abundance of free radicals that damage nearby cells.

Ordinary nutrients, particularly the minerals iron and copper, can react precipitously with oxygen to create free radicals, which is why the body ordinarily protects its stores of these metals from coming in contact with cells (the molecule hemoglobin, which carries oxygen in red blood cells, for example, keeps iron snugly sheltered in a molecular cage that prevents the formation of free radicals). If iron becomes detached from its safe harbor, as occurs with trauma or injury, it can set off a chain reaction of free radicals that can pose a greater risk to a person than the initial wound. Even more dangerous may be the iron overload caused by eating iron-fortified foods and vitamin-mineral supplements. This insidious form of iron supplementation (iron is intentionally added to many commercially made food products, such as breads, packaged cereals, and vitamin supplements) may overload the body's capacity to handle the mineral, resulting in health problems, such as heart disease, stroke, and brain and nerve damage.

Researchers have recently suggested that one reason why premenopausal women are less susceptible to heart disease and stroke than are men is that women lose a great deal of iron through menstruation and hence carry much less iron in their blood. Mounting evidence now reveals that cholesterol carried in the blood becomes "toxic" (causes damage to the arteries with a consequent buildup of plaque) when it is transformed (oxidized) by free radicals and that this free-radical chain reaction may damage arteries and set the stage for heart attacks and strokes.

Scientists now know that cigarette smoke (especially side-stream, or secondhand smoke), air travel (exposure to cosmic rays at high altitudes), a high intake of polyunsaturated fats (their molecular structure renders them highly susceptible to free-radical formation), X rays, air pollution, ordinary metabolism, and even exercise all produce free-radical chain reactions in the body. Given the ubiquity of free radicals, what can you do to protect your mind and body against these molecular terminators?

Antioxidant Smart Synergy

Antioxidant nutrients behave like nutritional smart bombs. They zone in on free radicals and entrap them, thereby minimizing the damage they do.

You can release the power of smart antioxidant nutrients only when you understand that each one helps magnify the power of the others contained in the Eat Smart, Think Smart antioxidant plan. The interaction of the antioxidants in the plan amplify its ability to neutralize free radicals. In some cases, one antioxidant can actually renew another antioxidant used up while quenching free radicals. Vitamin C, for example, can reenergize an oxidized molecule of vitamin E. Likewise, many of the B-complex vitamins provide antioxidant benefits in their own right and work as coantioxidants by permitting other antioxidants, such as beta-carotene and vitamin E, to keep scavenging and defusing free radicals much longer than would otherwise be possible.

This mutual-protection and magnification effect among various antioxidants, known as *synergy,* provides powerful protection against free-radical damage and even affords protection against the generation of free radicals by antioxidants themselves. Old or improperly stored vitamins and minerals can actually oxidize, or turn rancid, essentially creating the very toxic free-radical compounds that they're supposed to squelch!

Vitamin C, for example, can oxidize into a toxic substance, DHA (dehydroascorbic acid). Vitamin E can turn into tocopherol quinone, an extremely toxic compound. Beta-carotene can oxidize into a pernicious substance that can damage cell membranes.

All too often, these and other antioxidant supplements can go bad in the bottle if stored under damp, hot, or brightly illuminated conditions. That's why I recommend purchasing antioxidants from reputable manufacturers (a good sign is that they've been in national distribution for at least ten years), storing them in a cool, dark, and dry place and *always* taking them in concert with each other (see also sources listed in Appendix I). The principle of synergy requires that if you take vitamin C, you must also take vitamin E, beta-carotene, and B-complex vitamins (some of which behave like antioxidants) to help reconstitute the antioxidants that would otherwise be sacrificed as they perform their job as free-radical quenchers.

The Eat Smart, Think Smart Suggested Antioxidant Formula

The quick way to benefit from the Eat Smart, Think Smart antioxidant plan is to take an antioxidant nutrient formula. For maximum free-radical protection take this formula two to three times each day with meals. Here are the ingredients (amounts listed are for an entire day):

- Beta-carotene: 25,000 IU
- Vitamin E (mixed tocopherols): 800 IU
- Vitamin C (calcium ascorbate): 2 g
- Ascorbyl palmitate: 100 mg
- Vitamin B_1: 25 mg
- Vitamin B_2: 25 mg
- Vitamin B_3 (niacinamide): 120 mg
- Vitamin B_5 (pantothenic acid): 250 mg
- Vitamin B_{12}: 100 mcg
- Folic acid: 800 mcg
- Inositol: 100 mg
- Zinc citrate: 30 mg
- Copper (coated gluconate): 2 mg
- Selenium (selenomethionine and selenate forms): 200 mcg
- L-glutathione: 500 mg
- L-methionine: 250 mg
- L-taurine: 250 mg
- Inositol: 100 mg
- Coenzyme Q_{10}: 30 mg

> Persons with Wilson's disease (an inherited condition characterized by excessive copper storage) should not take any nutritional supplement containing copper without first checking with a physician.

The suggested antioxidant formula contains the most important antioxidants your brain needs to shield it from free-radical damage. You can obtain substantial antioxidants from vegetables, fruits, and whole grains, but foods alone cannot supply anywhere near the megadoses of antioxidants and vitamins found in the antioxidant formula or similar nutrient-mix products sold in health food stores and by mail order (it's really the only practical way to get all the smart nutrients just listed, see Appendix I for suppliers of these products). Thus, although it's important to enjoy an antioxidant-rich diet, you should also supplement your diet with antioxidants to create a shield against free radicals to prevent brain aging.

A number of antioxidant formulations that approximate the formula listed here are sold throughout the United States in health food stores, pharmacies, and by mail-order companies. Two of my favorite formulations are these:

- Maxi-Life CoQ$_{10}$ (Twin Laboratories; available in health food stores): one of the best-designed antiaging formulas for maximum free-radical protection; available in capsules or powder.
- Life Extension Mix (Life Extension Foundation; see Appendix I for mail-order information) contains an extensive complement of antioxidants and exotic nutrient cofactors; available in capsules or powder.

You may wish to supplement these antioxidant formulas with additional nutrients, especially calcium (none of the formulas contain the amount recommended by nutrition experts—800 to 1,200 mg per day—to help prevent osteoporosis).

If you follow the Eat Smart, Think Smart antioxidant protection plan, outlined in the next section, the antioxidant formulas just mentioned will provide most of the nutrients required to prevent premature brain aging.

Smart Antioxidants for Your Mind

Here is a list of the key antioxidant smart nutrients and vitamin cofactors that form the core of the Eat Smart, Think Smart antioxidant protection plan. This miniplan will minimize the free-radical damage that occurs each day as the brain uses oxygen to create energy and to synthesize and metabolize neurotransmitters. The dosage ranges are those used in commonly available commercial antioxidant formulations and individual supplements.

VITAMIN C. The brain has special vitamin C pumps that concentrate the antioxidant ten to fifteen times the concentration carried in the blood for good reason: Of all the known antioxidants found in the body, the most powerful is vitamin C. Vitamin C is superior in its free-radical quenching ability to other water-soluble antioxidants, such as uric acid; bilirubin; and sulfur-containing amino acids like cysteine and methionine. Recent research has shown that although the antioxidants that mix well with fats (including vitamin E, beta-carotene, and coenzyme Q_{10}) can reduce (but not eliminate) the damage from free radicals in the brain, they are unable to prevent the initiation of free-radical damage. Only vitamin C is powerful enough to intercept the chemicals (oxidants) that start the free-radical chain reaction. Vitamin C traps free radicals that escape all other free-radical defense systems in the body. It is the only antioxidant found in the body that is capable of completely protecting blood lipids against peroxidative damage from cigarette smoke, thus strengthening the argument that vitamin C supplementation is essential for all who breathe cigarette smoke, either directly or indirectly.

Vitamin C does not work alone and should be viewed as only one link (albeit an essential one) in the antioxidant chain. It has been shown to work closely with another antioxidant, glutathione (a "tripeptide," which is composed of three amino acids). Glutathione, not vitamin C, is probably the pivotal water-soluble antioxidant *inside* the cell (since vitamin C is water soluble, it cannot penetrate each cell's lipid, or fatty membrane).

Although vitamin C cannot scavenge free radicals within the lipid region of brain neurons, another antioxidant, vitamin E, which is located in the lipid portion of cell membranes, helps suppress free-radical attacks, being consumed in the process. When vitamin C is present in sufficient quantities, free radicals are quenched for a longer period and as efficiently as if *additional* vitamin E were present. Furthermore, the rate of the free-radical destruction of vitamin E can be decreased by the presence of vitamin C. Vitamin C thus acts as a synergist with vitamin E because it helps regenerate vitamin E after it has been "exhausted" in its role of quenching free radicals. Vitamin C is a safe, inexpensive, and nontoxic antioxidant and provides one of the brain's most powerful defenses against free-radical damage. *Dosage: 1,000–3,000 g per day.*

Vitamin C–rich Foods

Black currants	Oranges
Broccoli	Papayas
Brussels sprouts	Peppers (green, sweet red, chili
Cabbage	peppers)
Collards	Potatoes
Grapefruit	Spinach
Kale	Strawberries
Kiwi	Tomatoes
Lemons	Watercress

ASCORBYL PALMITATE. This fat-soluble form of vitamin C has been used for years as an antioxidant in animal feed, yet it has only recently been used as a nutritional supplement. Because regular vitamin C is water soluble, it can't penetrate cellular walls; it works only outside the cell's membrane (extracellularly). However, ascorbyl palmitate's fat solubility allows it to penetrate the cell wall (thus working intracellularly). We're covering all bases by taking both forms of it. Although no studies have yet been conducted to discern the antioxidant potential of ascorbyl palmitate in the brain, it is theoretically possible and quite likely that this fat-soluble form of vitamin C can protect the brain and central nervous system against premature aging induced by free radicals. *Dosage: 100–200 mg per day.* (Note: ascorbyl palmitate is synthesized in the laboratory and is not found in foods.)

VITAMIN E. Vitamin E is generally acknowledged to be nature's most effective fat- and free-radical quenching antioxidant for cells and organs that are rich in lipids (fats and oils). That's good news for anyone who wants to prevent premature brain aging, since the brain contains one of the highest concentrations of unsaturated fatty acids of any organ in the body. One study revealed that vitamin E plus the trace element selenium prevented age-related changes that normally occur in brain cells. These changes were defined by measuring the accumulation of pigmented waste materials that typically accumulate with age. These waste materials have been implicated in causing brain disorders, such as the loss of neural function and senility. It is interesting that we tend to absorb and store more vitamin E the older we get. A study at the University of California at Irvine, for example, revealed that as we age, we tend to absorb more vitamin E in the lymphatic fluid after digestion, making vitamin E more widely available to the whole body.

A study conducted at Texas A & M University examined red blood cells from laboratory animals that were fed a diet deficient in vitamin E. It found that new red blood cells from vitamin E–deficient rats behaved like old red blood cells from healthy rats, as determined by their ability to function properly. The data suggested that oxidation that was due to vitamin E deficiency was the cause of the premature aging of red blood cells. Since red blood cells carry oxygen (via hemoglobin) to the brain and central nervous system, an insufficient intake of vitamin E can deprive the brain of optimal oxygenation. When oxygen leaks back into the "strangled" areas of the brain, a process called "reperfusion" can set off free-radical chain reactions that can severely damage brain neurons.

With the widespread use of diets that are high in complex carbohydrates, getting enough vitamin E from foods may be more difficult than ever, since many people now embrace low-fat diets that restrict the use of vitamin E–rich foods, such as vegetable oils. Vitamin E supplements that contain a variety of structurally related vitamin E molecules called vitamers (alpha, beta, gamma, and delta forms) offer a wider degree of antiaging protection than do those that contain just one vitamer. Its easy to spot the former type of vitamin E supplement by looking on the label for the identifying term "mixed tocopherols." This term is your assurance that you are purchasing the right type of vitamin E that will afford you optimal protection from free radicals. *Dosage: 400– 1,200 IU.*

Vitamin E–rich Foods

Almonds	Sunflower oil
Corn oil	Sunflower seeds
Cottonseed oil	Walnuts
Filberts	Wheat germ
Peanut oil	Whole-grain flour
Safflower oil	

BETA-CAROTENE. Beta-carotene is the primary form of vitamin A contained in the plant kingdom. It is sometimes called pro-vitamin A because it performs no vitamin A activity until it is transformed by the liver into active vitamin A (one molecule of beta-carotene is split into two molecules of vitamin A; because the body converts beta-carotene to vitamin A only as needed, vitamin A toxicity is not possible). It is not the vitamin A activity of beta-carotene, however, that gives the molecule its antioxidant power. Beta-carotene's real value as an antiaging smart nutrient derives from its ability to neutralize a pernicious form of oxygen (called singlet oxygen), contained in cigarette smoke, air pollution, and other environmental toxins, that can cross the blood-brain barrier and prematurely age the brain. Although there is no known toxicity to beta-carotene, people who drink lots of carrot juice or take large doses of beta-carotene in nutritional supplements may experience a harmless, orangelike skin discoloration that disappears once the amount of beta-carotene intake is reduced. *Dosage: 15–30 mg per day* (equivalent to 25,000–50,000 IU potential vitamin A activity).

Beta-carotene-rich Foods

Apricots	Kale
Asparagus	Mustard greens
Broccoli	Pumpkin
Cantaloupe	Spinach
Carrots	Squash (winter, summer)
Endive	Sweet potatoes
Iceberg lettuce	

VITAMIN B_1 (THIAMIN). This jack-of-all-trades B vitamin is intimately involved in the metabolism of all nerve and brain cells, and some of the highest concentrations of this vitamin are found in these cells. Vitamin B_1 is a coantioxidant that works with other antioxidants, such as vitamin B_6 and vitamin E, to neutralize free radicals. It prevents the abnormal bonding between amino acids, called cross-linking, which tends to age everything from skin to brain cells, and helps the brain turn glucose and oxygen into energy. B_1 also has a special function in counteracting the effects of two environmental pollutants: cigarette smoke and alcohol. *Dosage: 25–80 mg per day.*

Thiamin-rich Foods

Brewer's yeast	Rice bran
Chick-peas	Rice, brown
Kidney (beef)	Salmon
Kidney beans	Soybeans
Liver (beef)	Sunflower seeds
Navy beans	Wheat germ
Pork	Whole-grain flour

VITAMIN B_2 (RIBOFLAVIN). This B vitamin causes the urine of supplement users to turn a distinctive designer-yellow color. Its primary role in the brain is twofold: to help the enzyme glutathione reductase make the potent antioxidant glutathione (discussed later) and to participate in energy production. B_2 helps recycle oxidized glutathione back to a reduced state in which it can detoxify free radicals. Strict vegetarians may be at risk of underconsuming B_2, since the main dietary sources are dairy products and meat. *Dosage: 8–25 mg per day.*

Riboflavin-rich Foods

Almonds	Chicken
Brewer's yeast	Kidney (beef)
Dairy products (cheese, milk, yogurt)	Wheat germ

VITAMIN B$_3$ (NIACINAMIDE). Vitamin B$_3$ is essential for the production of the brain's neurotransmitters and its use of carbohydrates for energy. It can be synthesized in the body from the amino acid tryptophan. Hundreds of enzymes in the body require some form of niacin, including those involved in the metabolism of protein and carbohydrates. One form of vitamin B$_3$, niacin, can cause a variety of undesirable conditions, including skin flushing, heart palpitations, peptic ulcer, and abnormal glucose tolerance and can react with medications, causing undesirable drug-nutrient interactions. That is why it is important to take this form of vitamin B$_3$ under a physician's guidance. The niacinamide form of vitamin B$_3$ does not cause the undesirable side effects noted with niacin. *Dosage (niacinamide): 30–125 mg per day.*

Niacinamide-rich Foods

Beets	Salmon
Brewer's yeast	Sunflower seeds
Chicken	Swordfish
Fish (especially halibut)	Tuna (white albacore)
Peanuts	Turkey
Pork	Veal

VITAMIN B$_5$ (PANTOTHENIC ACID). This powerful vitamin and antioxidant plays a central role in the production of intercellular energy in the brain and is required to synthesize brain neurotransmitters, such as acetylcholine. A deficiency of pantothenic acid can cause degeneration of the protective casing around the spinal cord, leading to paralysis; studies have shown that vitamin B$_5$ can help. It can also help protect against the damage to arteries caused by dietary cholesterol and has recently been shown to stimulate cells of the immune system. *Dosage: 50–250 mg per day.*

Pantothenic Acid–rich Foods

Blue Cheese	Meats, all kinds
Brewer's yeast	Peanuts
Corn	Peas
Eggs	Soybeans
Lentils	Sunflower seeds
Liver (beef)	Wheat germ
Lobster	Whole-grain flour

VITAMIN B$_6$ (PYRIDOXINE). This B vitamin is involved in the metabolism of amino acids and requires vitamin B$_2$ for conversion to an active form. This illustrates just one of many interrelationships among the B-complex vitamins, a fact that underscores the importance of taking dietary supplements that contain all members of this vitamin group. Vitamin B$_6$ aids in the breakdown of glycogen, the storage form of glucose, the primary fuel required by the brain.

Vitamin B$_6$ is required to prevent damage to arteries that can result from the consumption of high-protein diets. B$_6$ fights atherosclerosis by preventing a by-product of protein metabolism (homocysteine) from injuring the artery wall, leading to the formation of plaque.

Even though research has shown that people with the lowest blood levels of B$_6$ experience heart attacks at a rate five times greater than people with the highest blood levels of B$_6$, too much B$_6$ can lead to nerve damage. In 1983, the first report that excess pyridoxine could be toxic showed that several people who ingested above 500 milligrams per day (some people routinely took as much as 6,000 milligrams a day without any other vitamin supplements) began to suffer from peripheral neuropathy. The nerve damage was found to be largely reversible once the megadose of B$_6$ was discontinued. A review of the scientific literature reveals that most reports of B$_6$ toxicity occurred when doses of 1 to 6 grams were ingested *without* other B-complex vitamins that could have minimized the toxicity of vitamin B$_6$.

Data on the safety of pyridoxine (vitamin B$_6$) in published studies suggests that doses approaching 1 gram a day for a prolonged period can result in the development of sensory neuropathy. Doses up to 500 milligrams per day appear to be safe on the basis of reports of the administration of pyridoxine for periods ranging from six months to six years.*

The U.S. Department of Agriculture has defined a diet as deficient in B$_6$

* *Toxicology Letters*, 34 (1986), pp. 129–39.

if it contains less than 1.5 to 2.0 milligrams a day. It has estimated that 80 percent of Americans may be deficient in B_6. This estimate, coupled with the probability that it takes 50 to 200 milligrams of B_6 a day to reduce the risk of atherosclerosis significantly means that more than 90 percent of Americans may not be getting the optimal dose of B_6 needed to prevent stroke and heart attacks. Certainly, people who eat protein-rich diets containing animal foods, such as eggs, cheese, milk, beef, and pork, need to pay special attention to obtaining adequate vitamin B_6. Since it is impossible to consume enough foods each day to obtain 50–200 milligrams of B_6 (66 bananas or 19 pounds of calf's liver contain about 50 milligrams of B_6), the only way to ingest optimal amounts of B_6 is through supplementation. *Dosage: 25–80 mg per day.*

Pyridoxine-rich Foods

Avocados	Salmon
Bananas	Shrimp
Bran (wheat and rice)	Soybeans
Brewer's yeast	Sunflower seeds
Carrots	Tuna (white albacore)
Filberts	Wheat germ
Lentils	Whole-grain flour
Rice (brown)	

VITAMIN B_{12} (CYANOCOBALAMIN). Vitamin B_{12} can actually be manufactured by microorganisms that normally inhabit the intestines with the help of vitamin B_2 and B_3. It is required for DNA synthesis and prevents anemia, which can decrease the amount of oxygen delivered to the brain. Elderly people tend to lose their ability to absorb vitamin B_{12} because of decreased levels of hydrochloric acid in their stomachs and the synthesis of a gastric-binding protein required for absorption. The sole source of vitamin B_{12} in nature is synthesis by microorganisms, and the vitamin is not found in plants unless they have been contaminated by microorganisms. The usual dietary sources of vitamin B_{12} are meats, milk and milk products, seafood, and poultry. *Dosage: 100–400 mcg per day.*

Vitamin B_{12}–rich Foods

Beef	Fish (especially flounder,
Cheese (blue and Swiss)	herring, mackerel, sardines,
Clams	and snapper)
Eggs	Milk and milk products

FOLIC ACID. Like vitamin B$_{12}$, folic acid is required for the synthesis of DNA. It also depends on vitamin B$_{12}$ to be reutilized by the body. Folic acid is required for the conversion of a toxic by-product of ordinary protein metabolism to a beneficial amino acid (the conversion of the amino acid homocysteine to the antioxidant amino acid methionine). Folic acid has recently been shown to prevent neurological deformities during fetal development, such as neural tube defects, in women who took folic acid supplements around the time of conception. *Dosage: 400–800 mcg per day.*

Folic Acid–rich Foods

Barley	Lentils
Beans (most types)	Liver (calf's)
Brewer's yeast	Oranges
Endive	Peas
Fruits (almost all)	Rice (brown)
Chick-peas	Soybeans
Green, leafy vegetables (almost all)	Sprouts
	Wheat germ

L-CARNOSINE. L-carnosine, which is available only from animal foods, works as part of a team of antioxidants, with vitamin C; the B-complex vitamins; beta-carotene; vitamin E; selenium; and the sulfur-containing amino acids, L-cysteine and L-methionine. L-carnosine is a potent "package" of two biochemically active amino acids that control or regulate at least thirteen important functions in the body.

L-carnosine performs impressive antioxidant activities as a potent scavenger of singlet oxygen, a devastating free radical found in air pollution and secondhand cigarette smoke. Another type of free radical known as the hydroxyl radical (produced during exercise, after eating a high-fat diet, and infection, for example) can be quenched if L-carnosine is present in high-enough concentrations. L-carnosine has been shown to be effective during the reestablishment of blood flow (reperfusion) after an artery closure, such as occurs in the brain during a stroke. *Dosage: 100 mg per day.*

L-carnosine-rich Foods

Eggs	Meat (all types)
Fish (all types)	Milk

COENZYME Q$_{10}$. Also known as ubiquinone (from the words "ubiquitous" plus "quinone"—a type of chemical-ring structure) (hereafter referred to as CoQ) is found throughout the animal and plant kingdoms. Although this compound takes various forms, the one found in humans and most higher animals is classified as CoQ, coenzyme Q$_{10}$. CoQ possesses the properties of a true antioxidant, much like vitamins E and C. Its main role is the production of energy in each brain cell, although it acts as a cell-membrane stabilizer (protector) against free radicals. The energy-producing actions of CoQ are intimately linked to vitamins B$_2$ and B$_3$, yet another reason why the full spectrum of antioxidant smart nutrients should be taken together. The richest dietary sources of CoQ are polyunsaturated oils, such as soybean oil. Monounsaturated oils, like olive oil, contain moderate amounts, while saturated fats, including those found in coconut oil, contain none. Beef, chicken, and some fish (albacore tuna and mackerel, for example) contain appreciable amounts, as do some nuts (roasted peanuts and walnuts).

In addition to obtaining some CoQ from plant and animal foods and the bacterial breakdown of plant-derived nutrients called bioflavonoids, the body ordinarily manufactures CoQ under normal conditions. CoQ is synthesized by the body from the amino acids L-tyrosine and L-methionine and shares a common synthetic pathway with cholesterol.

Concentrations of CoQ in the brain are influenced by exposure to stress, cold, and illness and are affected by hormone concentrations, drugs, and physical activity. Lowered levels of CoQ have been reported in people with diabetes, periodontal disease, muscular dystrophy, and cardiovascular disease and those who are undergoing total parenteral nutrition (a hospital feeding procedure in which a liquid diet is fed to patients by intravenous injection).

CoQ is technically classified as a nonvitamin nutrient, which means that it can be obtained from the diet or be manufactured in the body. Dietary supplementation may be desirable, however, under conditions that create CoQ deficiency as were just described.

CoQ can help protect against fat-induced "peroxidation"—the process whereby oxygen combines with unsaturated fats to create free radicals—and is equal to vitamin E in this respect, except that vitamin E is destroyed in the protective process, whereas CoQ is not. CoQ can prevent and cure some symptoms of vitamin E deficiency.

The most thoroughly studied benefits of CoQ have been in the area of cardiovascular disorder, such as stroke and heart attack. CoQ has been found to protect against damage caused by oxygen deprivation to tissues. Blood and tissue concentrations of CoQ have been shown to be depressed in humans with cardiovascular disease, with the magnitude of the deficiency corresponding to the severity of the disease. *Dosage: 10–90 mg per day.*

COQ-rich Foods

Beef	Spinach
Peanuts	Tuna (white albacore)
Sardines	

SELENIUM. One of the most potent anticarcinogens in the antioxidant smart-nutrient arsenal, selenium works best with vitamin E in protecting the body against free radicals. As part of the enzyme system glutathione peroxidase, selenium helps protect cells against lipid peroxidation. Two forms of selenium—selenate and selenomethionine—have been shown to be absorbed effectively and to be used by the body. Selenate helps to elevate levels of glutathione peroxidase rapidly, whereas selenomethionine increases levels of the antioxidant in the tissues. *Dosage: 100–400 mcg per day.*

Selenium-rich Foods

Bran (wheat and rice)	Kidney (beef)
Broccoli	Liver (calf's)
Cabbage	Milk products
Celery	Mushrooms (most types)
Chicken	Onions
Cucumbers	Wheat germ
Egg yolk	Whole-grain flour
Garlic (fresh)	

ZINC. Zinc is a mineral involved in many enzyme systems in the brain, including superoxide dismutase, a powerful antioxidant system that neutralizes a particularly destructive form of oxygen (zinc works in tandem with the mineral copper in this regard). Zinc also serves as a potent cell-membrane stabilizer against free-radical damage. Taking excess zinc or consuming zinc-rich foods, such as lamb, organ meats, shellfish, and nuts, can interfere with the body's ability to absorb copper, so care must be taken to include both minerals in any nutritional supplement formula. The brain contains substantial quantities of zinc, which may help prevent the accumulation of environmentally acquired lead. *Dosage: 15–30 mg per day.*

Zinc-rich Foods

Beef	Pork
Bran (wheat and rice)	Soybeans
Egg yolk	Sunflower seeds
Fish (especially herring)	Turkey
Lamb	Wheat germ
Molasses (black strap)	Whole-grain flour
Oysters	

COPPER. Copper is an essential mineral that can actually serve as a pro-oxidant, or free-radical initiator, causing the type of cellular damage that leads to cerebrovascular disease. However, it can be consumed in low-enough doses to protect against oxidative damage as part of superoxide dismutase, an enzyme complex with zinc. Vitamin C and zinc tend to serve as safety factors, preventing the body from absorbing excess copper. Oysters, other shellfish, beans, peas, lentils, wheat germ, and copper cookware and utensils provide the richest sources in the diet. *Dosage: 1–2 mg per day.*

Persons with Wilson's disease (an inherited condition characterized by excessive copper storage) should not take any nutritional supplement containing copper without first checking with a physician.

Copper-rich Foods

Barley	Nuts (Brazil, cashews, filberts,
Lentils	walnuts)
Molasses (blackstrap)	Peanuts
Mushrooms	Wheat germ
Oatmeal	

INOSITOL. Inositol is a sugarlike molecule found in high concentrations in the brain that serves as a brain cell–membrane stabilizer. In various forms, it is present in plant and animal foods (in plants inositol is called phytic acid). *Dosage: 250–500 mg per day.*

Inositol-rich Foods

Beans (most types)	Nuts (most types)
Cantaloupe	Oatmeal
Chick-peas	Pork
Fruits (most citrus, except	Rice (brown)
lemons)	Veal
Lentils	Wheat germ
Liver (calf's)	Whole-grain flour

GLUTATHIONE. Glutathione is a stable tripeptide (composed of three amino acids) that contains the antioxidant sulfur-containing smart nutrient cysteine. Since pure L-cysteine can be degraded in the body into the potentially toxic product cystine (which may precipitate kidney stones), I recommend taking glutathione because it is not broken down into harmful substances. Glutathione is completely absorbed from the gastrointestinal tract and cannot crystallize in the kidneys. Just as important, it can be recycled in the body by certain enzymes. This smart nutrient protects against the cross-linking of proteins, which leads to the decline in function of each brain cell. L-cysteine can protect against many environmental toxins, including air pollution, cigarette smoke, heavy metals, and alcohol. It also functions as the effective portion of glutathione peroxidase, a free-radical-protection enzyme system that contains selenium. *Dosage: 250–500 mg per day.* Note: Glutathione is manufactured by the body from amino acids (protein) and is also available as a smart-nutrient supplement.

L-METHIONINE. L-methionine, which is available only from animal foods, is a sulfur-containing amino acid that serves as an antioxidant in the brain. It helps prevent the buildup of heavy metals, such as cadmium and mercury, in the brain and plays an essential role in the production of the brain neurotransmitter choline. *Dosage: 100–250 mg per day.*

L-methionine–rich Foods

Eggs	Milk
Fish (all types)	Poultry (all types)
Meat (all types)	

L-TAURINE. L-taurine is a nonessential antioxidant amino acid that functions as an electrical-charge stabilizer in the conduction of nerve transmission in the brain and nervous system. Even though it is synthesized in the body from the amino acid cysteine, L-taurine is absent from all plant foods. It reaches a high concentration in the developing nervous system, serves as a cell-membrane stabilizer, and contributes to the synthesis of the neurotransmitter glutamate. In this way, L-taurine serves as a depressant, limiting the synthesis of this excitatory neurotransmitter. Shellfish, lamb, and pork contain appreciable amounts of L-taurine, as do muscle meats. *Dosage: 100–500 mg per day.*

L-taurine–rich Foods

Eggs   Meat (all types)
Fish (all types)   Milk

5

Intelli-Sex

What could be sexier than a romantic, candlelit dinner with the right person? Sensuous lovers know how to use food as gastronomic foreplay—a culinary prelude to an evening's pleasure. Food is sensual stuff. But a romantic menu isn't sensual only because it tastes wonderful or looks good by candlelight. Your body's natural sex chemicals—dopamine, norepinephrine, androgen, and estrogen—are influenced by the actual foods you eat, not only by the romantic mood in which you eat them.

Nutrients have affected human sex drive for as long as there have been human beings. You may drive the newest-model car, wear the trendiest new fashions, and live in the most modern residence, but you still inhabit the body of a cave dweller. You respond to the same primitive drives and neurochemicals that moved your prehistoric ancestors to satisfy their carnal desires. When it comes to sex, we are all still driven by urges that whetted stone-age sexual appetites—fueled by the smart nutrients that our body turns into sex hormones and aphrodisiaclike chemicals.

Although most physicians regard substances that are claimed to enhance sexual desire or prowess as swindles perpetrated by quacks and charlatans (in 1982, the FDA declared that it could find no evidence to support the claims made by manufacturers of a number of alleged aphrodisiacs), evidence from research seems to indicate that there are at least a few genuine sexually stimulating nutrients and drugs. Despite lingering and widespread skepticism, a number of physicians, psychologists, and research scientists have acknowledged that the body does manufacture substances that have an aphrodisiaclike effect from smart nutrients.

In this chapter you'll learn everything you always wanted to know about smart nutrient "aphrodisiacs." First I'll give you a little historical background, exploring a few myths and corroborating some ancient folk wisdom. As you'll see, human beings have been benefiting from aphrodisiacs for thousands of years. Then you'll get a list of foods that especially affect sexual drive, mood, and performance, to help you construct your own erotic eating menus from the foods you like best. Next you'll learn what the sex-enhancing substances in your body and the nutrients you consume actually are and how they affect sexual performance. Finally, I'll tell you about the natural sexual stimulants that you can find in any health food store and give you two recipes for sex-enhancing smart drinks that you can create if you want to do so from scratch, designed specifically to enhance your sexual pleasure and experience in three main areas: increasing your sex drive, intensifying orgasm, and overcoming impotence.

Don't let anyone tell you there's no such thing as an aphrodisiac. In this chapter, you'll learn that there are quite a few. Not that everything touted as an aphrodisiac *is* one. Let's sort out the myths from the realities right now.

Sex and Foods: Fact and Fable

Throughout history certain foods have been associated with sexuality. In Renaissance Italy, for example, impotent men drank an elixir made from egg yolks, wine, butter, cinnamon, nutmeg, and sugar that they hoped would cure them. The Kama Sutra promised that eating pomegranates would enlarge the penis. As recently as fifty years ago, Chinese brides were advised to snack on peaches, figs, and other fruits associated with female fertility. Still other cultures have recommended dining on such exotic fare as tiger penises, kangaroo genitals, and white moss scraped from the skull of a corpse to fan the flame of sexual desire.

For centuries, and in almost every culture, fruits and vegetables that bear a physical likeness to either the male or female sex organs have been promoted as sexual aids. The Aztecs likened the avocado to the testicle (because of its shape) and refused to let maidens outside when the fruit was being harvested; Asians, Africans, and Philippinos endowed the phallic banana with mythical sexual properties; the Greeks did the same thing with carrots; Hindus saw the fig as representing both the vagina and the penis; and the Chinese saw peaches and apricots, with their provocative clefts and appearance, as sexual foods.

Not all foods considered aphrodisiacs come in the shape of sex organs, however. The ancient Greeks and Romans recommended eating large amounts of onions to improve sexual endurance, and Aristophanes prescribed garlic as a cure for impotence. Honey and eggs (to the ancient Egyptians as well as to many others); cacao (to the Aztecs); and later, chocolate (introduced by the Spanish explorer Hernán Cortés), all have been praised for their aphrodisiac qualities.

You may be tempted to laugh at some of these ancient beliefs, but don't laugh too long. Scientists have examined the nutritional content of many of these foods and discovered a basis for these long-standing beliefs and traditions. Bananas are rich in the mineral potassium, which is essential for the proper functioning of nerves and muscles. Carrots are an excellent source of beta-carotene, a form of vitamin A that helps control the production of sex hormones and vaginal secretions. Garlic and onion contain chemicals that can lower elevated levels of cholesterol in the blood, a cause of impotence. Eggs contain choline and essential amino acids, which are used to make neurotransmitters that are involved in the sex drive. Cacao and chocolate both contain an amino acid that similarly makes neurotransmitters that affect sex drive and libido. Figs and avocados contain niacin (vitamin B_3), which not only affects orgasmic pleasure, but lowers elevated blood cholesterol levels, a cause of impotence.

Obviously our forebears from around the world were on to more than they knew when they told us to eat avocados, chocolate, and onions. But what precisely are the nutrients in smart foods for sex, and how do they achieve their effects?

Two Groups of Smart Nutrients for Sex

There are basically two groups of nutrients that we'll look at more closely: first, the natural substances your body produces that have an aphrodisiac effect and second, smart nutrients that influence sex drive, erection, and orgasmic pleasure.

Your Body's Own Natural Aphrodisiacs

Here are a few examples of substances the body naturally produces that have been found to have a direct effect on sexual drive and performance, with a brief description of how they affect your body and how the body derives them:

Dopamine, made in the brain from the amino acid L-tyrosine, stimulates alertness, excitement, and sexual desire. The prescription drug L-dopa (used to treat Parkinson's disease) can increase the brain's production of dopamine, leading to increased sex drive.

Acetylcholine, the primary neurotransmitter of the parasympathetic nervous system, helps control blood flow to the genitals in women and men, heart rate, and blood pressure during sexual intercourse. It is manufactured from choline or lecithin, vitamin C, vitamin B_6, vitamin B_5, and zinc.

Norepinephrine is the primary neurotransmitter used by the sympathetic nervous system to stimulate the sex drive. It is made from the essential amino acids L-phenylalanine and L-tyrosine and vitamin C and vitamin B_6.

Nitric oxide, a gas made in the body, has recently been discovered to be essential for penile erection. A gas that acts as a neurotransmitter, it is active for only five to ten seconds and seems to control blood flow in and out of both the penis and women's genital tissue. The body makes nitric oxide from the amino acid L-arginine.

Estrogen, secreted by the ovaries and the adrenal glands (in both sexes), helps maintain the health of the vaginal mucous membrane, stimulates lubrication, and preserves tissue elasticity. Postmenopausal women who are undergoing estrogen-replacement therapy report an increase in sexual desire and drive. It is interesting to note that postmenopausal women who are sexually active secrete more estrogen than do those who are not; thus sexual activity can reduce the need for estrogen-replacement therapy to treat the side effects of menopause, such as vaginal dryness.

Progesterone, another sex hormone secreted by both men and women, is highest in women during the second half of their menstrual cycles (it stimulates the uterine lining in preparation for pregnancy). Low progesterone levels are thought to be related to the onset of premenstrual syndrome, or PMS. Progesterone has been tested in men as a hormonal contraceptive, and though it inhibited fertility, it also depressed the men's desire for sex.

VIP (vasoactive intestinal polypeptide) helps dilate the blood vessels in the sexual organs of both sexes. Some researchers believe that a deficiency of this neurotransmitter is a primary cause of organic impotence in men when a psychological cause is ruled out. Researchers are now focusing on treating impotence with direct injections of VIP.

Oxytocin, produced in the pituitary gland at the base of the brain, is involved in the muscular contractions during orgasm (it is secreted by the brains of both sexes during sexual climax). Oxytocin has been credited with promoting feelings of romance and nurturance.

As I've said, the production of these naturally occurring substances can be influenced and enhanced by the consumption of certain foods and smart supplements. This is especially the case with the second group of sex-enhancing nutrients: vitamins and minerals.

Smart Nutrients for Sex

Smart nutrients play an important role in sexuality, and their presence in smart foods provides a powerhouse of sexual potency for those who are smart enough to seek them out. Since vitamins and minerals and other nutrients are fragile—many are destroyed by cooking, metal pans, and light or are leeched out of foods during preparation—you may be getting less of these vital nutrients than you think. The following vitamins and minerals will help keep you in top sexual form. I've listed the latest RDA for each nutrient, so you can compare these values with those found in many commercially available antioxidant formulas (see chart 3.1). The RDAs—most of which are, in my opinion, worthless—change every four years or so and are designed, at best, to prevent *deficiency* diseases (such as scurvy, beri-beri, and pellagra), but have little relevance to maximum mental performance, life extension, and the overall prevention of degenerative diseases. Anyone who is familiar with the scientific literature is aware that most studies that have demonstrated the beneficial effects of nutrients (especially antioxidants) in humans have used *many, many times* the RDA for the majority of nutrients.

Thiamin (B_1) is essential for optimal nerve transmission and energy production throughout the body—which means it's essential for sex. (Chronic alcohol use predisposes one to thiamin deficiency.) Natural food sources include beans, peas, lentils, raw nuts, soybeans, whole-grain cereals and breads, seeds, peanuts, and yogurt. *RDA: 1 mg minimum.*

Niacin (B_3), in addition to combating depression, insomnia, anxiety, and fatigue, helps dilate blood vessels that are important for maintaining penile erection in men and clitoral erection in women. It helps the body synthesize sex hormones, such as estrogen and testosterone, and, like thiamin, helps the body convert foods into energy. Niacin can lower elevated blood cholesterol levels, a cause of impotence, but the most common form of vitamin B_3, niacinamide, cannot do so.

Niacin may cause temporary skin flushing, burning, itching, redness, and heat which usually last no more than 15–30 minutes. This reaction is generally harmless and can be minimized by taking niacin supplements on a full stomach. All people, including those taking antihypertensive (high blood pressure) medications, those with gout, diabetes mellitus, or a history of liver disease, gallbladder disease, peptic ulcer, arterial bleeding, or acanthosis nigricans, should consult with a physician before taking niacin supplements.

Pantothenic acid (B_5) is popularly known as the stress vitamin because laboratory tests show that animals that are exposed to environmental or mental stress survive longer when their diets are rich in pantothenic acid. Vitamin B_5 helps the adrenal glands manufacture steroid hormones and has been used to treat PMS. Vitamin B_5 is found in poultry, beef, eggs, beans, potatoes, broccoli, cabbage, cauliflower, and molasses. *RDA: no recommended dosage; 4–7 mg are suggested.*

Pyridoxine (B_6) (commonly found in vitamin supplements as pyridoxal-5-phosphate) is required for the transport and metabolism of amino acids that serve as precursors to the synthesis of neurotransmitters, such as dopamine and norepinephrine, that are involved in the sex drive. Birth control pills and estrogen-replacement therapy can lower the levels of B_6 in the body. Foods that are rich in this vitamin include eggs, red meat, bananas, carrots, cantaloupe, wheat germ, and sunflower seeds. *RDA: 2 mg for men, 1.6 mg for women.*

Cyanocobalamin (B_{12}) helps the body manufacture hemoglobin, the oxygen-carrying molecule found in red blood cells (low levels of vitamin B_{12} can result in a type of anemia that can cause, among other things, a loss of sex drive). Vitamin B_{12} is essential for proper brain and nerve development and for DNA synthesis. Strict vegetarians need to supplement their diets with vitamin B_{12} because it is found in appreciable amounts only in animal food sources. Vitamin B_{12} is found in muscle and organ meats, fish and shellfish, milk and milk products, eggs, and seaweed (contaminated with vitamin B_{12} from microorganisms). *RDA: 2 mcg.*

Folic acid is required for the production of energy, the synthesis of nucleic acid, the division and replication of cells, and the formation of red blood cells. Birth control pills and hormone-replacement therapy can deplete levels of folic acid in the body. Recent research has shown that folic-acid supplementation, around the time of conception, can help prevent birth defects of the central nervous system (one of the most important nutritional discoveries, in my opinion, of the twentieth century). Folic acid has also been used in the treatment of cervical dysplasia. It is found in such foods as green leafy vegetables, root vegetables, organ meats, tuna, salmon, whole grains, wheat germ, cheese, and citrus fruits. *RDA: 200 mcg for men, 180 mcg for women.*

Vitamin C participates in the synthesis of hormones that are involved in sex and fertility: androgen, estrogen, and progesterone. In addition to aiding in growth, tissue repair, and bone healing and offering widespread protection against free-radical damage throughout the body and central nervous system, vitamin C is vital to the formation of connective tissue (collagen), which helps keep skin supple, elastic, and youthful looking. It is found in citrus fruits and tomatoes; green leafy vegetables, such as cabbage; and broccoli. *RDA: 60 mg; 100 mg suggested for smokers.*

Vitamin A and beta-carotene are involved in cell growth, vision, protection against free-radical damage to the lungs and mucous membranes, the production of healthy sperm, and the maintenance of a properly functioning thyroid gland. Vitamin A also helps regulate the synthesis of the sex hormone progesterone. Vitamin A is found in two forms, preformed vitamin A and pro-vitamin A, or beta-carotene. Carotene is a pigment found in vegetables, such as yams, carrots, yellow squash, and pumpkin. Carotene is converted by the body to active vitamin A only when needed, so it is relatively nontoxic, even when taken in large amounts. Vitamin A is made from carotene in the bodies of other animals, which are subsequently ingested by humans in foods, such as liver, milk, and eggs. Other foods that are high in carotene include tomatoes, broccoli, and green leafy vegetables. *RDA: 1,000 RE for men, 800 RE for women.*

Vitamin E, often referred to as the sex vitamin, is a powerful antiaging antioxidant that protects cell membranes from free-radical damage and is required for the synthesis of hormones and hormonelike substances known as prostaglandins. Food sources of this vitamin include vegetable oils, nuts, seeds, beans, whole grains, egg yolks, wheat, spinach, fruits, peas, and asparagus. *RDA: 10 mg for men, 8 mg for women.*

Anyone taking large doses of vitamin E should consult an ophthalmologist to make sure they don't have retinitis pigmentosa (half of
all those who develop RP have no idea that they're at risk because it's
a recessive trait). More information on RP can be obtained from the
RP Foundation (800-683-5555). Those people scheduled for surgery
who take vitamin E supplements should inform their physician prior
to surgery because vitamin E can prolong bleeding times.

Zinc, in terms of sex, primarily affects men, because it is required
for the production of testosterone and proper functioning of the
prostate gland. It has been shown to help manage prostatitis and
some cases of impotence. Food sources of zinc include oysters, beans,
peas, lentils, pumpkin, sunflower seeds, and spinach. *RDA: 15 mg for men,
12 mg for women.*

Magnesium participates in the synthesis of sex hormones and has
been used to treat PMS and menstrual cramps. It is vital to proper
muscle and nerve functioning. Foods rich in this mineral include
meats, fish, dairy products, avocados, apples, apricots, figs, peaches, beets,
and whole grains. *RDA: 350 mg for men, 280 mg for women.*

Manganese is a trace mineral that is important for the production
of sex hormones, such as androgen and estrogen, and neurotransmitters that modulate the sex drive, such as dopamine and
norepinephrine. Good food sources include apples, apricots, leafy green
vegetables, whole grains, beets, and nuts. *RDA: none; 2–5 mg recommended for adults.*

Two Recipes for Sexual Success:
Orgasm and Impotence

Now that you've learned what the smart sex nutrients are, how they work,
and what foods to find them in, here's how to use them to the best
advantage, concentrating on two important areas: orgasm and impotence.

For orgasm: the orgasm-enhancing smart-nutrient formula U4EA supplies your cells and central nervous system with the essential chemicals
it requires to trigger and sustain sexual climax. *For impotence:* the

Power-Up formula will provide the necessary chemicals required by the body to enhance, maintain, and sustain an erection.

These two formulas—or smart-nutrient miniplans—have helped my clients enjoy a fuller and more vital sex life. I'll tell you how to make them yourself from their component parts—vitamins, minerals, and nutrients you can find in most vitamin or health food stores. (Note: if you want to remind yourself what these nutrients do, look them up in the two previous sections on the body's natural aphrodisiacs and vitamins and minerals. I'll explain what a particular nutrient is and what it does in the following section only if I haven't covered it already.)

Use a potent multivitamin-mineral formulation, such as CoQ_{10} Maxi-Life (Twin Laboratories) or Life Extension Mix (Life Extension Foundation) each day to supply the necessary nutritional cofactors that will help these two formulas achieve their maximum effectiveness (see Appendix I for information on ordering).

Smart Sex Miniplan 1: The U4EA Formula for Orgasm

The ecstasy of sexual climax, or orgasm, has inspired volumes of poetry and great literary epics and has changed the course of history (in all likelihood, it was more than Helen of Troy's face that launched a thousand ships). The following smart nutrients may not help you achieve anything quite so grandiose or historic, but they can enhance one of nature's most sensual gifts. The nutritional components of the U4EA formula are available at health food stores or through most of the sources listed in Appendix I. You can make it yourself from the following ingredients. As I said before, the majority of people will suffer no side effects from these supplements, but if any cautions listed do apply to you, take heed.

Directions: Mix one serving of choline cocktail and take niacin, histidine, and carnosine capsules at the same time, approximately thirty minutes before sex.

Choline Cocktail (Twin Laboratories) stimulates the release of the sex-related neurotransmitters norepinephrine and dopamine (from the green tea in the formula which contains caffeine, a substance that sensitizes the brain to the stimulatory effects of norepinephrine) and the synthesis of acetylcholine (from choline, which is converted to acetylcholine, the neurotransmitter related to sexual performance and arousal); both are sex-related neurotransmitters. (You can make your own choline cocktail using the recipe on p. 26.) *Dosage: 1 serving.* (See choline warning, page 22; L-phenylalanine warning, page 27.)

Niacin (vitamin B_3) causes the release of histamine from cells, the chemical responsible for the uniquely pleasurable sensation of orgasm. *Dosage: 25 mg.* (See niacin warning, page 74.)

L-histidine, an essential amino acid, provides the raw material for the synthesis of histamine, the chemical released at the moment of orgasm in the sexual organs and trunk of the body, responsible for flushing and pleasurable sensation. *Dosage: 500 mg.*

People taking antihistamines or those with severe allergies should avoid taking histamine supplements.

L-carnosine is an amino acid that serves as a storage molecule for histamine, the chemical responsible for the physical sensation of orgasm. *Dosage: 250 mg.*

Smart Sex Miniplan 2: The Power-Up Formula: Smart Substances That Keep It Up

Smart nutrients offer hope for men who have difficulty achieving or maintaining an erection. Sexual stimulants have been used for thousands of years to address this universal sexual problem, but so much myth and misconception surround their use that it is hard for the layperson to separate fact from fiction.

Smart nutrients and drugs, including nonprescription plant extracts and herbs, supply the body with the essential chemicals that stimulate, control, and regulate erections. Recent research has uncovered the biochemical and neurologic basis for erections.

You can purchase the ingredients for Power-Up at your local health food store or from the sources listed in Appendix I.

Directions: Mix one serving of choline cocktail and take on an empty stomach approximately thirty minutes before sex. Use L-arginine–rich foods (pick your choices from foods in the list in Chart 4.1 that contain 2–4 grams of L-arginine) each day if possible.

Choline cocktail (use Twin Lab's Choline Cocktail made with fructose and xylitol, or make your own using the recipe on p. 26). NutraSweet (brand name, Equal) is broken down into L-phenylalanine, an essential amino acid that is converted to the sex-drive neurotransmitter dopamine in the brain.

L-arginine is the only known nutrient from which the neurotransmitter nitric oxide (responsible for penile erection) is made. This essential amino acid, found in protein foods, such as chicken and turkey, is on the FDA's hit list for reclassification as a drug. Chart 4.1 contains a list of L-arginine–rich foods that you can enjoy to obtain a satisfactory supply of this erection-inducing essential amino acid. *Dosage: 2–4 g, two hours before sex.*

> L-arginine can cause an outbreak of herpes virus in sensitive individuals who are already infected with the virus. In addition, recent research has shown that large doses of L-arginine may accelerate the growth of preexisting cancer cells.

CHART 4.1
L-arginine–rich Foods

Milligrams		Quantity
4,147	Spirulina	3½ ounces
2,641	Soybean nuts, dry roasted	½ cup
2,414	Beef (center loin)	3½ ounces
2,391	Beef (top loin)	3½ ounces
2,086	Turkey (white meat without skin), roasted	3½ ounces
1,993	Chicken (white meat without skin), baked	3½ ounces
1,777	Crayfish, steamed	3 ounces
1,680	Beef liver, pan fried	3½ ounces
1,673	Corned beef (cured), canned	3½ ounces
1,658	Ground beef (extra lean), baked	3½ ounces
1,584	Clams, steamed	3 ounces
1,561	Kidneys (pork), braised	3½ ounces
1,539	Pumpkin, roasted	1 ounce
1,522	Tuna (bluefin), baked	3 ounces
1,522	Lobster (northern), steamed	3 ounces
1,509	Shrimp, raw	3 ounces
1,500	Crab (blue), steamed	3 ounces
1,499	Duck (without skin), roasted	3½ ounces
1,496	Beef kidneys	3½ ounces
1,493	Chicken liver	3½ ounces
1,476	Mussels (blue), steamed	3 ounces
1,458	Split peas, boiled	1 cup

Milligrams		*Quantity*
1,437	Crab (Alaska king), steamed	3 ounces
1,416	Cottage cheese, low fat, 2 percent fat	1 cup
1,408	Tongue (beef), simmered	3½ ounces
1,391	Salmon (coho, poached	3 ounces
1,389	Salmon (sockeye), poached	3 ounces
1,380	Lentils, boiled	1 cup
1,369	Chickpeas (garbanzos), boiled	1 cup
1,360	Ham (cured, lean), raw	3½ ounces
1,358	Crab (Alaska king), raw	3 ounces
1,357	Halibut (Atlantic), poached	3 ounces
1,356	Tuna (white albacore), canned in spring water	3 ounces
1,350	Tuna (white meat), canned in oil	3 ounces
1,340	Trout (rainbow), baked	3 ounces
1,337	Snapper, broiled	3 ounces
1,326	Pine nuts (pignoli), dried	1 ounce
1,323	Tofu, raw	½ cup
1,291	Swordfish, broiled	3 ounces
1,289	Ham, cured	3½ ounces
1,283	Haddock, smoked	3 ounces
1,277	Cottage cheese (low fat, 1 percent fat)	1 cup
1,264	Grouper, broiled	3 ounces
1,255	Pike, northern, broiled	3 ounces
1,221	Navy beans, canned	1 cup
1,215	Ocean perch (Atlantic), broiled	3 ounces
1,204	Pompano (Florida), broiled	3 ounces
1,202	Sea bass, broiled	3 ounces
1,199	Mackerel (Spanish), broiled	3 ounces
1,195	Great northern beans, canned	1 cup
1,193	Broadbeans, boiled	1 cup
1,190	Whitefish, smoked	3 ounces

Case Study: Smart Nutrients, Sex Drive, and Healing a Broken Heart

Several years ago I found myself sitting at the bedside of a world-famous movie director—I'll call him David to protect his true identity—who was hospitalized for a heart attack. Our long-term plan was to get him on his feet and prevent this type of problem from happening again. Smart nutrition can do that. But the objective that day was *survival,* and survive he did.

Human nature allows us to be elated by a victory (such as cheating the grim reaper) one day and feeling cheated the next week as the novelty of the miracle wears off and the reality of recovery sets in (what I call the "Why me?" syndrome). After a while it's not enough just to be alive, with health restored; you want to start living *well*. With my help, I was certain David would. Once he recovered, his pressing problem was of a sexual nature because a "post–heart attack depression" had taken its toll on his sex life.

After reducing his blood cholesterol to safe levels and starting him on a regular exercise program, I formulated a smart nutrient plan to help elevate his mood and mental energy, restore confidence in his physical abilities, and rekindle his sex drive. The rest fell into place.

About eight weeks after he followed my advice, David sent me a gift with a note to phone him. On the phone he said, "There is nothing in the world like making love to a beautiful, talented, and intelligent woman and feeling up to the challenge of pleasing her in every way. For the first time in years, I'm confident about my physique and sexual stamina. Actually, I've *never* felt this way before. Youth isn't all it's cracked up to be!"

Confidence *is*. David was able to rise to the occasion (so to speak) with a younger-looking body and a more youthful mind-set because of his smart-nutrient regimen. In this case, the older man got the girl, and now, by all accounts, they have a thriving two-career celebrity marriage, five years old and going strong.

6

Sweet Dreams:

The Smart Way to Get a Good Night's Sleep

You've seen how smart nutrients can wake up your brain, but can they help you go to sleep? If you are one of millions of people who grapple with sleepless nights, the smart nutrients I call "smart sleepers" may be the answer to your bedtime prayers.

For most healthy people, difficulty falling asleep is probably due to the stress and worry that accompany daily life. Faulty sleep patterns are also a common disorder of aging. Uncontrollable thoughts and concerns can easily keep people awake for hours past their normal bedtimes; others may awaken inappropriately in the middle of the night and have difficulty falling back to sleep.

Scientists who study sleep have identified patterns of chemical changes that occur in the brain and the body during sleep. The smart nutrients I'll tell you about in this chapter are used by the brain to induce and control sleep, so you can enjoy a good night's sleep without resorting to prescription medications that are so often abused and lead to dependence and drug overdose.

First, I'm going to tell you about the brain's sleep system that responds to the smart nutrients called sleepers. Then I'll tell you how sleepers work, safely and effectively, to put you to sleep and how to take them either in food or as supplements. Finally, I'll show you how to mix up your own sleep-inducing cocktail that can help you enjoy a drug-free night's sleep.

Sleeplessness is sometimes caused by an underlying medical disorder that may require the help of a physician. Before you try any of the smart nutrients in this chapter, check with your physician to ensure that your sleeplessness is not due to a serious illness.

Smart Sleepers: A Safer Alternative to Drugs

Smart sleepers act on the same sleep-inducing areas of the brain as do prescription and over-the-counter sleep aids, but they can help you get to sleep without posing the risk of serious side effects.

The class of sedative-hypnotic drugs—loosely known as sleeping pills or downers—are widely used in low doses to calm people during the day and in higher doses to help them sleep at night. Millions of people take sleeping pills every night and can't fall asleep without them. Every year, an untold number of people suffer health problems or die as a result of sedative-hypnotic abuse.

Barbituric acid, the grandfather of all sleeping pills, was discovered at the end of the Civil War. Since then, a number of derivatives have been marketed throughout the world. The first barbiturate sleeping drug, called barbital, was marketed in 1903, followed by phenobarbital in 1912.

Some barbiturates are metabolized slowly and remain in the body for weeks. Others are metabolized more quickly (in six to seven hours). These are the barbiturates most people take to fall asleep. They can make people feel and even look drunk, cause hangovers, and kill by putting the brain's respiratory center to sleep. They can also easily lead to addiction and unpleasant withdrawal syndromes, which are marked in some cases by convulsions and even death.

It is especially dangerous to mix barbiturates and alcohol because their depressant effects are additive. An ordinarily safe amount of alcohol or dose of barbiturate taken separately could be lethal if mixed.

Over-the-counter sleeping pills, used as directed, are somewhat safer than are prescription sedative-hypnotics, but are not without untoward effects. Like other pharmaceuticals, their abuse can lead to memory loss and hangover and can make driving or operating machinery hazardous. They can even cost you a great deal of money. Ivan Lendl, whose nutritional counselor I've been for a number of years, used a popular over-the-counter brand of sleeping pill to get to sleep the night before the 1990 U.S. Open Tennis finals. The next morning's hangover, and the consequent brain-dulling side effects of the sleep aid, may have cost him the championship.

People who use prescription or over-the-counter sleeping aids should be aware that these drugs are strong depressants that can cause unpleasant side effects and dependence and, when abused, even death. Smart-nutrient sleepers provide much safer and equally effective alternatives to prescription sedatives.

Sweet Dreams Are Made of These

Here's a list of smart-nutrient sleepers, followed by an explanation of how they work:

- L-tryptophan
- DMAE (dimethylaminoethanol)
- Vitamin B_1 (thiamin)
- Vitamin B_2 (riboflavin)
- Vitamin B_3 (niacinamide)
- Vitamin B_5 (pantothenic acid)
- Vitamin B_6 (pyridoxine)
- GABA (gamma-aminobutyric acid)
- Inositol

The best way to understand how these smart sleepers work is to learn how the brain's three sleep centers make use of them.

1. *The benzodiazepine system* is a brain neurotransmitter system that affects sleep. The well-known prescription sedatives Valium, Librium, and Dalmane all affect this system because their molecular structure "locks" onto cell membranes, thereby triggering the release of the brain's own sleep chemicals. One of these chemicals is GABA (gamma aminobutyric acid), which works in concert with the sugar inositol (found in nerve-cell membranes and muscle), and vitamin B_3 (niacinamide) to help lock onto and activate the benzodiazepine sleep system. The important difference between sleepers and prescription drugs is that sleepers are generally nonlethal in relatively large doses even if taken with alcohol. Barbiturates, in general, have a high potential for abuse with life-threatening consequences if mixed with alcoholic beverages.

2. *The cholinergic nervous system,* which is controlled by the brain neurotransmitter acetylcholine, helps control body movement, such as sleepwalking, tossing and turning, and general muscle activity, during sleep. As people age, there is a marked decline in the activity of the cholinergic system that can lead to poor sleep. The smart nutrients choline, DMAE, lecithin, vitamin B_5, vitamin B_6, and vitamin C can help optimize brain levels of acetylcholine (too much acetylcholine can cause excessive muscular activity, such as sleepwalking or sleep-disrupting body movements).

3. *The serotonergic system,* activated by the essential amino acid L-tryptophan is also involved in regulating sleep (serotonin initiates calmness and relaxation in certain areas of the brain). There is a nifty trick to getting L-tryptophan out of foods and into your brain to induce sleep that I'll tell you about in the following section.

Again, smart sleepers offer a much safer and, in most cases, equally effective alternative to potentially dangerous prescription sleep aids without the undesirable side effects that can hamper mental and physical performance. The Rockabye Formula that I'll tell you about shortly uses a combination of vitamins, other nutrients, and foods to get you a safe and restful night's sleep. But first, I want to tell you more about an important sleep-inducing amino acid, L-tryptophan, that you can get from ordinary foods. Since the FDA has banned the sale of L-tryptophan supplements (because a bacterially contaminated batch of L-tryptophan from Japan caused serious health problems in those who took the tainted pills), you'll need my guide to finding L-tryptophan in foods and to learn how to use it.

The Special Role of L-tryptophan in Sleep

In human beings, L-tryptophan is the raw material the brain uses to make serotonin, melatonin, and niacin (vitamin B_3). All three by-products of L-tryptophan metabolism can help you enjoy a good night's sleep. L-tryptophan thus plays a key role in helping regulate sleep-wake cycles in the brain.

Over twenty years ago, researchers at MIT demonstrated that when people eat a protein-poor, high-carbohydrate meal (such as spaghetti with tomato sauce), L-tryptophan from carbohydrate-rich foods goes right to their brains. The researchers discovered that compared to other amino acids, L-tryptophan has a unique advantage: Carbohydrates cause insulin secretion by the pancreas; insulin then clears all other amino acids from the blood that compete with L-tryptophan for entry to the brain, leaving only L-tryptophan, which is then shuttled across the blood-brain barrier into the brain. Once in the brain, L-tryptophan is converted to serotonin, giving the pasta lover a sense of satiety, a feeling of well-being, and the ability to drift off to dreamland (many antidepressant drugs also work by increasing levels of serotonin in the brain).

Dietary L-tryptophan increases the amount of REM (rapid eye movement) sleep, a stage of sleep that involves dreaming and deep rest. It also stimulates the production of melatonin, a neurohormone that helps control sleep-wake cycles. When too little L-tryptophan gets into the brain, melatonin synthesis declines, leading to the increased probability of nightmares and, consequently, a poor night's sleep (melatonin, in turn, causes the release of a brain chemical called vasotocin, which is also involved in REM sleep). Since melatonin secretion tends to decline with age, it's not surprising that elderly people have more trouble falling asleep and sleep less than they did in their youth.

Most people eat 1 to 1.5 grams per day of dietary L-tryptophan. Two to four grams of L-tryptophan have been used clinically to reduce the time required to fall asleep when taken one to two hours before retiring, but even 500 milligrams (one-half gram) of L-tryptophan can induce sleep. Because of its scarcity in food and severe competition with other amino acids for entry to the brain, it is difficult to ensure that the intake of L-tryptophan is high, even when protein intake is low. Stress, which makes it difficult to fall asleep, complicates the matter because it tends to lower levels of L-tryptophan in the body (cortisol, a hormone released in response to stress, is responsible for this effect). Stress thus creates a vicious cycle of sleeplessness by depleting the very amino acid that the brain needs to fall asleep.

The L-tryptophan Nightmare

In the summer and fall of 1989, a newly described medical syndrome occurred in epidemic fashion across the United States. Evidence quickly linked the syndrome to the ingestion of L-tryptophan supplements from one specific manufacturer in Japan.

Many people who had the misfortune to purchase contaminated L-tryptophan suffered from a variety of neuromuscular symptoms. The occurrence of this health problem reached epidemic proportions, and by June 1990, at least 1,500 cases of the syndrome, called EMS (eosinophilic myalgia syndrome), including 26 deaths, had been reported nationwide.

Investigators subsequently identified a bacterial endotoxin as the contaminant in an otherwise harmless shipment of L-tryptophan. The FDA moved quickly to remove all L-tryptophan supplements from the marketplace, an action reminiscent of the Tylenol scare, in which all capsules were removed from stores until the source of the contamination in a relatively small number of bottles was found. Once the source of the contamination of the Tylenol bottles was discovered (a mentally deranged individual), the FDA permitted the sale of Tylenol once again. This was not to be the case with L-tryptophan.

The FDA has recently announced that it will seek to ban the sale of *all* amino acids, including L-tryptophan, and will reclassify them as drugs, even though all the foods we eat are chock-full of amino acids. It is interesting to note that the FDA permits physicians to prescribe L-tryptophan and other amino acids for people who are ill. Hospitalized patients, including infants, are routinely given L-tryptophan and other amino acid supplements to *restore* their health with no apparent side effects.

People have used L-tryptophan supplements for years to help them get to sleep safely and effectively. Before the single contaminated batch was imported from Japan, no known deaths were ever attributed to L-tryptophan. In contrast, thousands of health problems are reported every year in people using prescription sedatives, especially when alcohol is used concurrently. L-tryptophan is not dangerous when used with alcohol, yet the FDA refuses to permit the sale of this beneficial amino acid, while it sanctions the sale of more harmful sleep aids.

Food Science to the Rescue

Just because it's illegal to sell L-tryptophan in the United States (L-tryptophan is available over the counter in Mexico and Europe) doesn't mean it's against the law to eat it in foods. Necessity is the mother of invention, so why not use a little food science knowledge to enjoy the sleep-inducing benefits of L-tryptophan, legally? Here's how:

Timing. You can get L-tryptophan into your brain quickly and efficiently if you eat low-protein L-tryptophan-rich foods one to two hours before retiring and two to three hours after dinner.

Minimize your protein intake. Protein-rich foods, such as dairy products, eggs, poultry, seafood, and meats, all contain large amounts of amino acids that compete with L-tryptophan for entry to the brain. This competition effectively blocks much of the L-tryptophan from reaching the brain in sufficient amounts and in time to put you to sleep. Protein-rich foods tend to wake up your brain because they contain large amounts of L-phenylalanine and L-tyrosine, two essential amino acids that stimulate the production of the neurotransmitter norepinephrine. Norepinephrine promotes arousal and mental activity, precisely what you don't need or want as you retire for the evening.

Choose carbohydrates. Sugars and starches cause the pancreas to secrete insulin, a powerful hormone that facilitates the entry of amino acids from the blood into cells. Insulin, however, does not affect L-tryptophan to the extent that is does other amino acids, so more L-tryptophan is left in the blood to be carried to the brain. The lack of competition from other amino acids allows L-tryptophan to enter the brain unobstructed.

Pick foods rich in L-tryptophan. Here's the difficult part: Most foods are so low in L-tryptophan and so high in competing amino acids that they're useless in boosting levels of L-tryptophan and the neurotransmitter serotonin that is made from it in the brain. There are, however, several foods and food combinations in which the ratio of L-tryptophan to other competing amino acids is high: bananas, dry-roasted sunflower seeds (an especially rich source), milk (skim milk will work just as well as whole milk), and baked potato (For the suggested amounts of these and other L-tryptophan–rich foods, see Chart 6.1). If you want a tasty L-tryptophan–rich bedtime snack, don't miss the Banana Custard recipe in Chapter 9 or the Lights Out (L-tryptophan Hot Toddy) in chart 6.3.

CHART 6.1
Selected Food Sources of L-Tryptophan

Milligrams	Food	Amount
929	Seaweed, spirulina	3½ ounces
164	Pumpkin (roasted)	1 ounce
115	Milk (whole, low-fat, or skim)	1 cup
99	Sunflower seeds (dried)	1 ounce
77	Potato, baked with skin	1 medium
77	Tomato soup made with skim milk	1 cup
49	Shredded wheat	1 ounce
48	Seaweed, kelp (kombu-tangle), raw	3½ ounces
48	Turnip greens (boiled)	½ cup
27	Collards (boiled)	1 cup

Smart Sleeper Nutrients

GABA and the Benevolent Bs

GABA it provides the brain with a ready-made chemical that can activate benzodiazepine sleep receptors and gently induce sleep. As a brain neurotransmitter (manufactured in the body from the amino acid glutamate, vitamin B_6, and vitamin C), it helps put the brakes on an overactive mind.

GABA is an amino acid supplement that is currently sold in health food stores and pharmacies. (Note: since the FDA may attempt to remove GABA from the market and reclassify it as a drug, it's a good idea to know which smart nutrients, just mentioned, you need to take to stimulate GABA synthesis.) GABA seems to work well in concert with vitamin B_3 (niacinamide) because this vitamin attaches to the same type of benzodiazepine receptor in the brain as it does. By taking GABA with niacinamide (and vitamin B_6, which assists in the synthesis and transport of GABA), you can apparently amplify the sleep-inducing effects of GABA. Food sources that are rich in niacinamide include beef liver, brewer's yeast, chicken, halibut, peanuts, pork, salmon, sunflower seeds, tuna, and turkey.

Inositol, often considered part of the B complex of vitamins (although it is not a vitamin), is a sugar found in muscles and cell membranes. It acts as a cell-membrane stabilizer (by neutralizing free radicals) and seems to facilitate the sleep-enhancing effects of GABA and niacinamide; some studies indicate that it can also perform as a mild antianxiety agent. Inositol can be purchased as a nutritional supplement and is found in the following foods: beans, calf's liver, cantaloupe, chick peas, lentils, nuts, oatmeal, pork, brown rice, wheat germ, and most whole grains.

Other members of the B-complex family that promote a good night's sleep include vitamins B_1 (thiamin), B_2 (riboflavin), and B_5 (pantothenic acid), all available as supplements. Thiamin is vital to proper brain and nerve metabolism and can be found in beef liver, brewer's yeast, whole wheat flour, chick-peas, kidney and navy beans, pork, brown rice (bran portion), salmon, dried sunflower seeds, and wheat germ. Riboflavin helps preserve the integrity of the nervous system and aids in the release of energy from food. Good food sources include almonds, brewer's yeast, chicken, beef kidney, and wheat germ.

Activating Your Brain's Cholinergic System with Choline

Choline chloride, lecithin, and DMAE are unique smart nutrients that help supply the brain with the raw material (choline) to make acetylcholine, a neurotransmitter that controls the brain's cholinergic nervous system. This system helps regulate bodily movements, such as sleepwalking and limb movements, during sleep. Acetylcholine synthesis also requires vitamin B_5, vitamin B_6, and vitamin C. DMAE is available as a nutritional supplement in powder, capsules, or liquid form (be sure to store it in a cool, dark place). The suggested common dosage is 100 milligrams a day. Choline- and lecithin-rich foods include cabbage, calf's liver, cauliflower, caviar, egg yolks, chick-peas, lentils, soybeans, and split peas. Vitamin B_5 can be found in brewer's yeast, corn, lentils, lobster, meats (all kinds), peas, soybeans, sunflower seeds, wheat germ, and whole grains.

Persons with gastric ulcers or a history of ulcers should use choline supplements only with the consent of a physician because choline may increase the production of stomach acid. Choline supplements should not be used by persons with Parkinson's disease or by those who are taking presceiption anticholinergic drugs.

The Rock-a-Bye Formula

The Rock-a-Bye Formula gives your brain what it needs after a full day's work—a full night's sleep. You can purchase the individual ingredients to this formula in health food stores and vitamin shops and make it yourself (see list of ingredients in Chart 6.2). This formula is designed to be used with the Lights Out Hot Toddy recipe (see Chart 6.3). Lights Out provides an inexpensive and readily available source of the FDA-banned amino acid L-tryptophan. For optimal results, take the Rock-a-Bye Formula with the Lights Out Hot Toddy one hour before bedtime.

CHART 6.2
Rock-a-Bye Formula

• One B-complex vitamin capsule (containing at least 10 mg of each B vitamin)	
• GABA	250 mg
• Inositol	100 mg
• Choline chloride	100 mg

All ingredients are available in capsules as separate nutrients. Take 1 hour before retiring with the Lights Out Hot Toddy recipe (Chart 6.3).

This is a quick and inexpensive way to get the essential amino acid, L-tryptophan, into your brain. Lights Out combines the L-tryptophan in skim milk and bananas with simple and complex carbohydrates found in those foods plus pure honey. Insulin, secreted in response to carbohydrates, drives all competing amino acids from the blood, leaving the L-tryptophan behind to enter the brain, where it is used to manufacture serotonin, a neurotransmitter involved in sleep.

1 cup skim milk
2 tablespoons honey
1 medium banana

1. Heat milk in saucepan until hot: add honey and stir
2. Add honey-milk mixture to blender and blend with banana until smooth.
3. Top with cinnamon and nutmeg and drink one hour before retiring.

7

Secrets of Muscular Development:

Anabolic Smart Nutrients

Muscle-building smart nutrients can mimic the beneficial actions of muscle-building hormones, such as anabolic steroids, without their devastating side effects. Smart nutrients can also reduce the catabolism (breakdown) of muscle protein. By using the unique combination of anabolic and anticatabolic smart nutrients in the Muscular Development Formula that I'll tell you about shortly, you can achieve maximal gains in muscle mass (lean body mass).

Anabolic Smart Nutrients: A Safer Alternative to Steroids

Testosterone, thyroid hormone, growth hormone, and insulin are the primary anabolic hormones that occur naturally in the human body. Athletes, particularly those involved in bodybuilding and in sports that require strength, such as jumping, sprinting, and throwing, have sought to enhance muscular development beyond the capabilities of the body's natural anabolic hormones. Injectable synthetic anabolic steroids quickly became the drugs of choice for success-driven athletes, a choice that has killed and maimed countless competitors who have been foolish enough to flirt with disaster.

It's not nice to fool Mother Nature, but as my world-class athletic clients have learned, its perfectly fine to work *with* her. That's where anabolic smart nutrients can help. These muscle- and strength-building nutrients can safely and effectively stimulate anabolism (muscle growth), prevent muscle breakdown (anticatabolism), and increase muscular endurance (ergogenesis) at the same time.

Each of the anabolic smart nutrients I'm going to tell you about can work individually and in concert to help you develop your own muscle tissue to its fullest genetic potential. It doesn't matter if you work out at a local health club or at home (I work out at home each day on my LifeCycle) or compete on the center court at Wimbledon. Anabolic smart nutrients can help anyone develop healthy, sound muscles that look good and help you enjoy peak performance in any sport or physical activity. These nutrients and the Muscular Development Formula I'll tell you about shortly will provide you with the latest developments in research devoted to the science of peak human performance.

First, I'm going to tell you how a certain class of amino acids (the branched-chain amino acids) can influence the quality of muscular growth, strength, and energy. Then I'll reveal how several important but often overlooked nutrients (ornithine alpha-ketoglutarate, carnitine, carnosine, creatine, glutamine, and chromium) can enhance your body's anabolic drive. Finally, I'll tell you all about protein supplements: how to chose the safest and most effective ones and why and how they work to achieve optimal muscular development. Women who want shapelier (but not necessarily bigger) muscles will benefit from learning how to pick the proper protein. Men who want more muscular definition and/or muscular strength will discover how these anabolic smart nutrients can enhance the muscle-building ability of their own natural male hormones.

The Branched-Chain Amino Acids (BCAAs)

BCAAs—leucine, isoleucine, and valine—are so named because they posses branchlike side chains of atoms, much like the branches on a tree. These side chains, which are unique to each amino acid, are usually the active sites of each molecule—the portion involved in metabolic reactions. Approximately 35 percent of the essential amino acids found in muscle are BCAAs; BCAAs are essential amino acids because they cannot be manufactured in sufficient quantities (or manufactured at all) by the body and therefore must be obtained from foods. In addition to nutritional supplements, BCAAs can be found in such foods as turkey, chicken, beans, lentils, peas, and seafood (see Chart 7.1).

BCAAs increase protein synthesis and decrease protein breakdown in muscles and can be oxidized (burned) inside muscle cells as a source of energy known as adenosine triphosphate, or ATP. The body also converts BCAAs (especially leucine, the most active BCAA) to glucose (sugar) during exercise in an effort to maintain optimal levels of glucose in the blood. Leucine also promotes the release of growth hormone, thyroid hormone, and insulin, exerting an anabolic or growth effect through the endocrine hormone system. BCAAs are the smart nutrients for active people because they are versatile.

BCAAs: Muscular fuel. Leucine and, to a lesser extent, the other BCAAs are used by muscles for energy, especially during intensive and prolonged physical activity. Studies have shown that physical training can activate the ability of muscles to burn leucine and the other BCAAs for fuel. Some of the beneficial effects of exercise training are due, in part, to the improved ability of muscles to burn BCAAs.

CHART 7.1
Essential Amino Acids in Selected Foods
(in mg/gm of protein)

	Foods					
Amino Acid	Egg White	Soy Beans	Casein	Lactalbumin	Brown Rice	Fish
Isoleucine	51	45	54	55	40	47
Leucine	83	78	95	109	86	77
Lysine	66	64	81	97	39	91
Methionine and cysteine	64	26	32	52	36	40
Phenylalanine and tyrosine	94	81	110	79	91	76
Threonine	47	38	46	41	41	46
Tryptophan	16	13	16	17	13	11
Valine	76	49	67	69	65	61

Alanine for Sugar. Alanine (a nonessential amino acid) is the most active amino acid responsible for the maintenance of ideal glucose levels during exercise and accounts for about half the glucose made in the liver. BCAAs are involved in this process, known as the glucose/alanine cycle. Here, in simplified form, is how it works:

During physical activity, leucine uptake by muscle tissue markedly increases and results in two effects: (1) part of the leucine molecule is used to make alanine and (2) the remaining part of the leucine molecule is burned for energy in the muscles. The liver converts the newly made alanine to glucose (in a process called gluconeogenesis). The net result is that leucine is burned for energy in the muscles, and alanine, after conversion to glucose in the liver, is used as a fuel source in muscle tissues.

BCAAs indirectly increase anabolism by reducing a muscle's need to burn its own proteins during bodybuilding or strenuous exercise. Biochemists call this the protein-sparing effect of BCAAs. As we've seen, leucine sacrifices itself to provide energy in muscle tissue and to produce alanine, which is converted to glucose in the liver. Since your body prefers not to burn precious muscle proteins as fuels, Mother Nature has provided less wasteful alternative fuel sources to prevent muscle wasting.

BCAAs stimulate the release of several anabolic hormones, such as human growth hormone, thyroid hormone, and insulin. Many people believe that thyroid hormone is catabolic, rather than anabolic (that it burns up, rather than builds up). However, thyroid hormone actually increases protein synthesis in muscles and thus is considered an anabolic hormone in spite of its catabolic actions on fats and carbohydrates

BCAAS AND MUSCLE PROTEIN. BCAAs can prevent muscle protein from being metabolized for energy. The BCAAs (particularly leucine) prevent muscle protein breakdown in a variety of catabolic states, such as severe burns, bacterial infection, and trauma (leucine's anticatabolic action has been attributed to its metabolic by-product, keto-isocaproate). Bodybuilding and other types of strenuous physical activities all increase protein breakdown in muscle tissue. Thus strength athletes and burn victims share a common attribute: both need extra leucine to prevent muscle tissue catabolism, or breakdown.

The Branched-Chain Keto Acids (BCKAs)

BCKAs are actually ammonia-free sources of BCAAs; as such, they provide a less toxic source of muscular energy and anabolic nutrition for muscular development. BCKAs are both made from and converted to BCAAs. Thus, they can function as dietary substitutes for BCAAs (the body can convert about 35–50 percent of BCKAs to BCAAs).

BCKAs, like BCAAs, can increase lean body mass, boost energy production in muscle, and help remove ammonia, a toxic by-product of protein metabolism. Thus, BCKAs are similar to BCAAs with respect to muscular development and athletic performance.

Detoxification of ammonia is an important action of BCKAs. Ammonia buildup causes muscular fatigue and hampers the body's ability to synthesize proteins. Keto-isocaproate operates as the body's most effective ammonia scavenger, working with other smart nutrients, such as glutamine (the most abundant amino acid in muscle tissue) and alpha-ketoglutarate (a by-product of ordinary metabolism) in keeping ammonia in the body at safe levels. Bodybuilders and strength athletes, two groups of athletes who ordinarily consume large amounts of protein (from foods and nutritional supplements), release significant amounts of ammonia into their blood as a result of strenuous exercise. This ammonia must be removed, or their performance and health will suffer. You can use BCKAs to improve your level of athletic performance and muscular development as well.

Ornithine Alpha-Ketoglutarate (OKG)

OKG is a muscle-building nutritional supplement that has caught the attention of athletes over the past few years because of its anabolic and anticatabolic effects. Ornithine stimulates the release of growth hormone (its anabolic effect), and alpha-ketoglutarate prevents protein breakdown (its anticatabolic effect). The novel combination of these two nutrients seems to accomplish more than when each is administered alone.

The body can also convert OKG into BCAAs and BCKAs, as well as into glutamine and glutamate (both help detoxify the ammonia produced from protein metabolism). OKG can also promote the release of two anabolic hormones, insulin and growth hormone. Recent clinical trials have shown that OKG helps increase muscle tissue in people who are recovering from burns and injuries.

Glutamate is the precursor to glutamine, the most abundant amino acid in skeletal muscle. Glutamine has an anabolic effect on muscle and can increase glycogen (the storage form of carbohydrate energy in the liver). Glutamate is also involved in the conversion of BCAAs to BCKAs.

Finally, OKG can remove ammonia created during the breakdown of muscle proteins. It can thus serve as an ammonia receptacle, minimizing muscular fatigue during and after exercise.

One recent study involving bodybuilders revealed that supplemental ornithine increased serum growth hormone levels up to 400 percent. OKG also enhances the release of insulin in healthy people, as well as in those with catabolic conditions. ornithine alone does not promote the release of insulin; keto-isocaproate, the BCKA made from leucine, is probably the actual stimulus for the release of insulin.

Creatine for Muscle Energy

Creatine functions as a storage molecule for phosphate, the ultimate source of muscular energy (as ATP). Creatine exists in muscle as creatine-phosphate (CP). Recent research has shown that athletes can deplete their muscle stores of CP in a relatively short time; for example, CP levels dropped as much as 90 percent after a single 400-meter sprint in one study).

Five grams of creatine can produce a significant increase in the level of creatine in the blood—an amount that corresponds to the amount of creatine found in about 2½ pounds of meat. Since no one should consume that much meat (because of the excessive amounts of saturated fat, cholesterol, and protein it contains), athletes rely on creatine supplements to obtain this valuable adjunct to muscular energy.

Increasing the amount of CP through supplementation can increase the availability of metabolic energy to draw upon, especially during those athletic events that are of short duration and high intensity. Athletes can also use creatine supplements to train harder and longer, thereby increasing muscle density and mass.

Boron

Some evidence suggests that boron (a trace mineral) may be of value in raising testosterone levels. A recent study, in which participants took a boron supplement (3 milligrams per day) raised testosterone levels in postmenopausal women. Additional studies of boron supplements, especially their usage by bodybuilders, are needed before any definitive conclusions can be reached.

L-carnitine

L-carnitine promotes the burning of fat in the body and thus spares proteins and carbohydrates from being catabolized and used as muscular fuels. Hence, L-carnitine is an anticatabolic nutrient because it spares the breakdown of muscle tissue.

Anabolic steroids (synthetic derivatives of testosterone) tend to increase levels of carnitine palmitoyl transferase, the enzyme that uses carnitine to carry fats into mitochondria to be burned for energy. They appear to activate the carnitine-mediated fat transport system, which may account, in part, for the loss of subcutaneous fat that bodybuilders who use injectable steroids seek. Since L-carnitine supplements also activate this system—safely and effectively and without the toxic side effects associated with steroid use—they provide a sensible alternative to harmful drugs. *Dosage commonly used: up to 4 grams per day.*

L-carnosine

I have used the dipeptide (two linked or bonded amino acids) carnosine to help the world-class athletes I counsel heal from sports injuries, boost their endurance, stimulate their immune systems, and recover faster from grueling competition and intensive training. To my surprise, every coach, trainer, and sports-medicine physician I have talked to has displayed an ignorance of the manifold and remarkable effects rendered by this simple dipeptide.

Even though scientists have long known about carnosine (it was discovered at the turn of the century) research studies have revealed many of carnosine's beneficial properties, I rarely find anyone who appreciates its nutritional powers.

Carnosine contains the biologically active amino acids L-histidine and beta-alanine. Each amino acid performs important biological functions that I will discuss shortly. The fact that carnosine is highly concentrated in muscle tissue belies its important role in controlling muscle contractility (carnosine derives its name from the Latin word for meat, or flesh).

Carnosine also possesses impressive antioxidant activity. Because of its ability to deactivate free radicals, the great Biochemist in the Sky saw fit to place high concentrations of this antioxidant dipeptide in the crystalline lens of our eyes to help protect against cataracts. As was just mentioned, muscle tissue is richly supplied with carnosine, and research has shown that carnosine (the histidine portion is the active amino acid in this case) protects against exercise-induced free-radical damage to muscle tissue. Carnosine can thus prevent unnecessary muscle breakdown and soreness after intensive training.

Even though carnosine isn't directly involved in the synthesis of ATP, it is intimately involved in increasing the concentration of enzymes that allow ATP to supply muscles with the energy to contract. Here's a simple version of how it does so.

Skeletal muscles have filaments (actin and myosin) that must slide across each other for a muscle to work or contract. ATP is required as an energy source for this contraction. Specific enzymes split off a phosphate group from ATP (the "P" in ATP stands for the phosphate molecule—there are three of them—attached to the nucleotide adenosine—the "A" in ATP), which releases energy used for muscle contraction. That's where carnosine comes in. It helps to activate the enzymes that split the ATP molecule to provide muscles with the energy they need to contract. Bodybuilders and power lifters would be weaker than the weakest 98-pound weakling at the beach without their carnosine and ATP. Let Popeye have his spinach; I'll eat my carnosine.

Chromium Picolinate

Chromium, an essential trace mineral, acts as an anabolic nutrient, in concert with the anabolic hormone insulin. The biologically active form of chromium is called glucose tolerance factor (GTF)—a complex of chromium, nicotinic acid (vitamin B_3), and three amino acids: cysteine, glutamic acid, and glycine (the same amino acids found in the antioxidant L-glutathione). GTF potentiates the actions of insulin by increasing the binding of insulin to insulin receptors that are located in cell membranes. GTF thus increases the body's sensitivity to insulin, improving the hormone's anabolic effects on muscle.

A scientist at the U.S. Department of Agriculture developed a form of chromium called chromium picolinate (the mineral chromium combined with a substance ordinarily made in the liver that improves chromium absorption and biological activity). Chromium picolinate has proved to be more potent than other forms of the mineral in a number of recent studies.

Many people, especially athletes, don't get enough chromium through their diets: 90 percent of self-selected diets were below the suggested safe and adequate intake of up to 200 micrograms of chromium per day. Physical activity and physical trauma (such as damage resulting from bodybuilding) accelerate the loss of chromium, which can be further aggravated by eating high levels of sugar.

High-protein diets, so common among bodybuilders, also increase the production of "insulinlike growth factor-1" (IGF-1, also known as somatomedin C)—a hormone that mediates, in large part, the actions of growth hormone. As protein intake increases, so do levels of IGF-1 in plasma. Which brings us to the final anabolic nutritional stimulant.

Protein: Quality vs. Quantity

A basic rule of muscular development is *the higher the quality of the protein, the lower the quantity required to support muscle growth.*

Though you're probably not aware of it, the package labels on many of the foods you eat reflect this relationship between quality and quantity. The "%RDA" listed is based on the need for 45 grams of protein a day.

To understand the assessment of the quality of protein, it helps to think of an ideal amino acid profile—the "perfect protein"—in which each essential amino acid occurs in precisely the right proportion. That is, each gram of the protein contains just the right number of milligrams of every amino acid.

The pattern of amino acids is vital because it determines how well the protein is utilized. Take too much of some amino acids (relative to the ideal), and they will be wasted; take too little of even a single amino acid, and the value of the entire protein will be compromised.

The amount of an amino acid in excess of the ideal required for protein synthesis is not stored; it is rapidly degraded. The nitrogen from the protein is excreted, mainly as urea. The organic acids that remain are oxidized for energy or converted to carbohydrates or fat. Conversely, when the amount of an amino acid is less than the ideal required for protein synthesis, protein from muscles and vital organs is broken down to supply the body with the essential amino acids that are lacking in the diet. Ideal amino acid patterns for high-quality proteins have been established by the Food and Nutrition Board of the National Research Council (NRC) in the United States (see Chart 7.2).

CHART 7.2
NRC Ideal Pattern for High-Quality Proteins

Amino Acid	*Milligrams per Gram of Protein*
Histidine	17
Isoleucine	42
Leucine	70
Lysine	51
Sulfur-containing amino acids	26
Phenylalanine and tyrosine	73
Threonine	85
Tryptophan	11
Valine	48

Casein (the predominant protein in cow's milk) has been known as the "gold standard" for measuring the quality of protein, but as can be seen from Charts 7.3 and 7.4, fish protein, lactalbumin (from whey protein), and egg proteins are most biologically active, on the basis of the measurements—PER and biological value—for evaluating the quality of protein. The significance here is that strength athletes and bodybuilders need the highest-quality protein for maintaining lean body mass. Moreover, athletes need higher amounts of specific amino acids (BCCAs) notably L-leucine.

As is shown in Chart 7.1, lactalbumin contains greater amounts of L-leucine than do other high-quality proteins. Therefore, lactalbumin, or whey proteins (the predominant protein in mother's milk), may be the preferred source of protein for athletes and competitive bodybuilders. Fortunately for mom, many commercially marketed amino acid–based powdered drinks contain whey protein.

CHART 7.3
PER Values of Proteins*

Protein	PER Value
Egg	3.92
Fish	3.55
Lactalbumin	3.43
Whole milk	3.09
Casein	2.86
Soy meal	2.30
Beef	2.30
Rice	2.18

* PER is defined as weight gain per gram of protein fed to laboratory animals.

CHART 7.4
Biological Value of Selected Proteins*

Protein	Biological Value
Whey (lactalbumin)	104
Egg (whole)	100
Egg albumin	88
Casein	77
Beef	80
Soy	74
Rice	59
Beans	49

* The biological value is defined as the amount of absorbed nitrogen retained in the body.

As Chart 7.4 reveals, whey protein enjoys the highest biological value of any dietary protein. But what is not evident in the chart is that it also contains the highest levels of L-leucine and other BCAAs.

PICKING THE RIGHT FORM OF SUPPLEMENTAL PROTEINS. There are three main classes of protein supplements: whole proteins, peptide-bonded proteins (partially-digested proteins or those that are chemically processed by a process that simulates digestion), and free-form, or single amino acids. Peptide-bonded amino acids (pancreatic-digested protein or predigested proteins) are the most biologically active, whole proteins are intermediate, and free amino acids are the least.

The normal digestion of whole proteins, such as those obtained from foods or supplements, takes up to four hours, with some of the protein left unabsorbed. Thus, one disadvantage to using whole-protein supplements is that they are incompletely utilized.

Single amino acids (the so-called free-form aminos that are the current rage among bodybuilders) result in the poorest nitrogen retention and are therefore the least anabolic. Single amino acids have another drawback: They increase intestinal osmotic pressure, which can interfere with the absorption of all nutrients and lead to diarrhea and intestinal distress.

Peptides are the most anabolic form of dietary protein supplements, absorbed faster than either single amino acids or whole proteins. They cause the highest nitrogen retention and do not cause intestinal problems. Bodybuilders and strength athletes should look for products (there are dozens) that contain peptide-bonded amino acids for optimal muscular development.

Persons with psychosis, insomnia, kidney or liver disease, hypertension (high blood pressure) those taking prescription MAO (monamine oxidase) inhibitors, those with cancer (especially pigmented malignant melanoma), herpes virus infections, or pregnant or lactating women should not take amino acid supplements unless advised to do so by a physician.

Using the Muscular Development Formula

I developed the Muscular Development Formula (see Chart 7.5) to meet the demanding training schedule of Martina Navratilova. Later, when I started counseling tennis champion Ivan Lendl, I improved it to reflect the latest scientific findings in the area of muscular development. This formula uses current nutritional technology to mimic the beneficial effects of anabolic steroids without the harmful side effects. As always, you should check with your physician before you begin an exercise or strength-training program, to determine if there is any medical reason why you should not take any of the nutrients in the formula.

CHART 7.5
The Muscular Development Formula*

Nutrient	*Dosage*
L-glutamine	1–2 g
BCAAs or BCKAs	2–4 g
Chromium picolinate	400 mcg
L-carnitine	250–500 mg
L-carnosine	100–500 mg
Creatine	1–5 g
OKG	5–10 g

* The nutrients in this formula are commonly sold individually as tablets or capsules in various dosages. Each nutrient can be used alone, but for maximum benefit, all should be taken with lunch or dinner.

8

Smart Drugs

The study of smart drugs, or nootropics (from the Greek words for "toward the mind"), is currently one of the most exciting developments in pharmaceutical research. Nearly every large pharmaceutical company in the world (and many small ones) is testing at least one experimental nootropic drug for possible approval by the FDA.

As odd as it may seem, the FDA has no category for drugs that improve memory and cognition in healthy people. In fact, the FDA will approve a drug only if it can be shown to be effective in treating a disease! People who are already afflicted with senility or Alzheimer's disease can seek treatment from a handful of FDA-approved drugs currently on the U.S. market, yet those who enjoy excellent mental health and wish to prevent Alzheimer's disease and other mental afflictions must head south of the border or cross the Atlantic to purchase brain-boosting (and brain-saving) smart drugs.

Fortunately, many nootropics are available from Europe, Japan, and Mexico through mail-order companies (see Appendix I for addresses and phone numbers). These drugs, according to published research, appear to enjoy a level of safety that surpasses most other types of prescription drugs. This statement seems reasonable because most smart drugs are based on the molecular structure of smart nutrients, which are drug-free and have few harmful side effects.

The research and development of smart drugs is still in its infancy, and the level of sophistication in the design of smart drugs has not reached full maturity. Some smart drugs, such as Hydergine (ergoloid mesylates) and Eldepryl (deprenyl, selegiline) have been proved effective and relatively nontoxic in humans. Fortunately, both drugs are approved by the FDA and are available in the United States by prescription. This means that a physician may prescribe these drugs for *any* reason (even to help "de-age" an apparently healthy brain) even though the FDA has not approved them for the *prevention* of medical conditions, such as senility.

Smart drugs offer a relatively safe way to energize the brain, improve memory, neutralize free radicals, and prevent brain damage that can lead to impaired mental performance and premature aging. Newer and more effective smart drugs are currently being tested by most major pharmaceutical firms, and I predict that these compounds will become the new magic mental bullets of the next century, extending life expectancy and improving the quality of life, much like antibiotics did in the twentieth century.

People who are adverse to using drugs of any type can still obtain many of the benefits of smart drugs by using smart nutrient equivalents. In this chapter, I'll tell you about four important types of smart drugs that can improve your memory, mood, and mental energy and help fight the effects of brain aging. When applicable, I'll tell you which smart nutrients you can use to achieve the same type of results as the corresponding smart drug. Finally I'll tell you how to import your own personal supply of smart drugs into the United States. This method is not only legal but is fully sanctioned by the FDA. Most people are unaware that the FDA actually permits individuals in the United States to mail-order smart drugs (provided the drugs are legal in their country of origin) from international suppliers without a physician's prescription.

Smart Drugs: Legal for the Time Being

Since 1988, an FDA ruling has made it legal for individuals to import a three-month personal supply of smart drugs (and other medications) as long as the countries from which the drugs are ordered consider them legal and safe. The FDA made this ruling, known as FDA Pilot Guidelines Chapter 971, under extreme pressure from AIDS political action groups, which asserted that the then-current FDA policy denied people with AIDS access to drugs available abroad that could potentially save or prolong their lives.

Since this 1988 ruling, the FDA has, from time to time, detained various shipments of smart drugs in the United States because of alleged violations by suppliers of smart drugs. Although these violations are relatively rare, there is no guarantee that the FDA will not change its policy about the importation of smart drugs by mail and reverse it in the near future.

What Smart Drugs Do

Smart drugs promote maximum mental performance in four basic ways. First, they supercharge the brain with an optimal supply of oxygen and the raw materials it needs to energize its neurons and store and recall memories. Second, they shield the brain against free-radical damage and other toxic substances that can lead to permanent brain damage. Third, they help remove cellular debris, called lipofuscin pigment (the same aging pigment that causes "liver spots" on the skin), from the brain, which has been linked to neuron damage and decreased mental performance. Fourth, they supply the brain with raw materials to replenish its supply of neurotransmitters.

Oxygen plays a Jekyll-Hyde role in the brain: It energizes the brain to think and remember more clearly while it ironically promotes free-radical damage that can lead to a host of neurological disorders, such as senility and stroke. Nootropic drugs play a unique role among all drugs in that they both optimize the delivery and use of oxygen to the brain and protect the brain from the hazards of oxygen-induced free radicals.

Should You Take Smart Drugs?

Just the thought of taking drugs turns off some health-conscious people I know. Many people, including those who run the FDA, seem to associate drugs exclusively with illness, disease, and pain. It's quite understandable that they have this attitude because we've grown up in a society where the practice of medicine is based on curing, rather than preventing, illness. Healthy people don't need to take drugs, right?

Not necessarily. Nootropic drugs may eventually change the way many people, including those at the FDA, view drugs. Since many nootropics are derived from or are based on the molecular structure of smart nutrients, they do not cause the highly toxic side effects of many other types of drugs in most normal, healthy people. Although smart drugs are synthesized in the laboratory, their molecular structure is often based on naturally occurring compounds found in foods and plants that are "friendly" to the human body.

Don't get me wrong. Nootropic drugs, like all substances, including air and water, can be harmful. That's why it's always important to consult with a knowledgeable physician if you decide to use these or any other drugs.

Some nootropics have been shown to extend the life expectancy of laboratory animals significantly. There is every reason to believe that nootropics can do the same to humans as well. People who are suffering from the early stages of memory loss or senility or who have suffered certain types of brain damage may experience dramatic changes, or "awakenings," when they use one or more nootropics. And, of course, healthy people can benefit from the memory and energy-boosting effects of nootropics that have already been documented in the medical literature.

The cognition-enhancing effects of smart drugs have been measured in the laboratory, but many of their positive benefits can be found in anecdotal case reports. Although these individual results vary from person to person, they nevertheless suggest the strong possibility that a significant number of people may enjoy the same beneficial results. At the least, the large number of anecdotal success stories should stimulate more definitive research in this exciting area.

Many people who use smart drugs report improvements in the following:

1. mental energy, alertness, and ability to concentrate
2. feelings of well-being, elevation of mood, and alleviation of depression
3. the ability to memorize written material
4. verbal memory
5. creativity and productivity
6. sexual performance and enjoyment
7. alertness with less sleep

Of course, people who are already operating at or near maximum levels of mental performance will probably notice fewer benefits than will those who are just trying to make it through the workday on six hours of sleep. Therefore, most people will probably enjoy some degree of cognitive improvement and may help stave off the type of brain damage that leads to some forms of senility by taking nootropics. That should be of some solace to those of us who still can't figure out how to program a VCR.

Four Important Smart Drugs for Maximum Mental Performance

The FDA does not yet recognize the drug category of nootropics, or smart drugs. Although dozens of compounds that are prescribed and sold throughout the world can be classified as nootropics, only a handful have been widely tested in the United States and abroad. The four types of nootropics that I'll tell you about enjoy exceptionally low toxicity, yet demonstrate a measurable and positive effect on the vital areas of memory, mental energy, and brain antiaging.

Piracetam (Nootropil)

Piracetam is considered to be the first true nootropic drug. Since it was developed by UCB Laboratories in Belgium in 1972, almost all major pharmaceutical companies have created some form of nootropic drug based on the molecular structure of piracetam.

HOW PIRACETAM WORKS. Piracetam increases alertness and enhances memory by stimulating the cholinergic system of the brain, especially in the cerebral cortex. The cholinergic system uses the neurotransmitter acetylcholine, which is synthesized from the smart nutrients choline (or the structurally related compounds lecithin and DMAE), vitamin C, vitamin B_5, and vitamin B_6.

Piracetam exerts the following effects on the brain:

1. It stimulates an increase in the metabolic rate and energy level of neurons.
2. It shields the brain against free-radical damage from hypoxia (oxygen deprivation).
3. It protects against loss of memory from trauma and poisoning from environmental toxins, such as pesticides and air pollution.
4. It heightens memory and learning in healthy people, as well as in those who have already suffered a degree of memory loss.
5. It facilitates the transfer of information between the right and left hemispheres of the brain.

PIRACETAM: MEMORY AND LEARNING. Several recent studies have confirmed that piracetam enhances learning, memory, and overall mental performance. One study of human subjects revealed that the mental performance of middle-aged people who were in good overall health but complained of a noticeable degree of memory loss improved significantly after four weeks of taking piracetam (4.8 grams per day).

Humans are the only animal species that possess a two-sided brain. The left and right hemispheres of the human brain each control specific mental functions. The flow of information between the two hemispheres has been demonstrated to be absolutely essential for harmonious and optimally sympathetic mental activity. Piracetam has been shown to improve (and even increase) the flow of information between the right and left hemispheres of the brain.

The two brain hemispheres are connected by a group of nerve fibers called the corpus callosum. It is mainly through these nerve tracts of networks that information from one hemisphere is transmitted to the other. This bidirectional aspect of the human brain dictates that nerves from the eyes and ears, for example, cross over to the opposite side of the brain. Therefore, sights and words that are received by the right eye and ear, respectively, are perceived by the left side of the brain, and information that is presented to the left eye and ear is sent to the visual and hearing centers on the right side of the brain. Piracetam seems to enhance the connection between (to "superconnect") both sides of the brain via the corpus callosum.

PIRACETAM INCREASES BRAIN ENERGY. The production of cellular energy depends upon the systematic buildup and breakdown of ATP. Biological aging decreases the amount of ATP available for conversion into energy, particularly in brain and muscle cells. The decreased amount of ATP, in turn, weakens the enzyme-induced processes that trigger the release of energy within the cells. Thus, as most people grow older, they find it increasingly difficult to perform under mental and physical stress, especially for long periods.

Piracetam promotes the synthesis of ATP, the universal form of cellular energy, in the cerebral cortex and so facilitates the transfer of information between the two cerebral hemispheres and increases the synthesis of proteins in brain cells, which research has established that long-term memory depends on.

Integrated information processing is suspected to be an important element of the creative insight enjoyed by artists, musicians, writers, and scientists. Some researchers speculate that because piracetam facilitates communication between the left and right hemispheres of the brain, it may enhance artistic, creative, and intuitive impulses. Piracetam does not produce the side effects that many people experience with the use of other synthetic stimulants that affect the central nervous system (such as amphetamines and cocaine). Even large doses of piracetam do not produce sedation or changes in brain waves or have adverse effects on the circulatory or respiratory systems. No toxic side effects have been reported in the medical literature following administration of piracetam to humans.

Dosage commonly used: 1.6 to 4.8 g per day (in 2–6 equally divided doses).

Sources: Piracetam is available in Mexico and throughout Europe and can be mail-ordered from the sources in Appendix I. A number of U.S. pharmaceutical companies are currently testing piracetam-based drugs that show promise as memory enhancers.

Ergoloid Mesylates (Hydergine)

Of the 20,000 new substances that are produced annually in the pharmaceutical research laboratories of the world, the vast majority are modifications of a few types of active compounds that are already in use. Chemists employed by drug companies attempt these chemical modifications to produce new, patentable (thus profitable) compounds with similar and perhaps improved activity over existing pharmaceuticals. Smart drugs are no exception.

In 1950, Dr. Albert Hofmann, a research scientist employed by the Swiss drug corporation Sandoz Pharmaceuticals, discovered a drug based on an existing molecule found in nature (a fungus that grows on grains) that he named Hydergine. Hofmann, a pioneer in the area of drugs based on molecules in plants, would become more famous for another drug he synthesized, based on the same fungus, the "smart" drug of the 1960s known as LSD_{25}. It is Hydergine, of course, that is the more important and safer smart drug.

Hydergine is the most widely used smart drug available in the United States today. It acts in many ways to enhance mental capabilities and to slow down or reverse the aging processes in the brain. Among the major effects of this cognitive-enhancing drug are these:

1. It prevents free-radical damage in the brain.
2. It increases the blood supply to the brain.
3. It enhances brain metabolism.
4. It increases the delivery of oxygen to the brain.
5. It protects against brain damage during periods of insufficient oxygen supply, such as during a stroke or asphyxiation.
6. It slows the depositing of age pigment (lipofuscin, the stuff of which "age spots" are made) in the brain.
7. It improves memory and recall.

Hydergine is actually a mixture of three fungus-derived chemicals (all derived from *Claviceps purpurea*). The Sandoz Pharmaceutical Company harvests *Claviceps purpurea* from rye fields in Europe and then extracts the fungi and chemically modifies them into the form used in the Hydergine formula. Hydergine is thus not a completely natural drug but, rather, a semisynthetic one because of the chemical steps necessary to change the natural fungus molecules into their final form.

Sandoz originally introduced Hydergine as a treatment for senility (senile dementia). Since many of the symptoms of senility are caused by atherosclerosis and calcification of the arteries in the brain (which deprives brain cells of vital oxygen), Hydergine, which can improve the delivery of oxygen to brain neurons, was a likely candidate for an anti-senility drug. Accordingly, the FDA approved the use of Hydergine for the treatment of senility and related circulatory problems.

Research published over the past fifteen years has shown Hydergine to be a safe and effective treatment for senility. Most people who were studied showed the greatest improvement with higher doses of Hydergine (4.5 to 6 milligrams per day), although the FDA has specifically limited the approved dosage of Hydergine to 3 milligrams per day (in Europe the approved dosage is 9 milligrams per day). Studies of humans have shown that the higher dosage levels are more effective. It is important to note that even at the higher dosage, there were no serious side effects.

Although Hydergine produces significant cognitive improvements in people who are suffering from senility, it does not produce miracles. Many people experience only a small amount of improvement in mental function, especially those with advanced senility. Hydergine is of greater benefit to people with mild to moderate mental deterioration, especially when Hydergine therapy is initiated soon after a medical diagnosis has been made.

Even though the FDA has approved Hydergine for the treatment of senility and cerebrovascular insufficiency (poor blood circulation to the brain), physicians in many other countries prescribe it for use in healthy people to increase intelligence, memory, and recall and to prevent the free-radical damage to the brain that can lead to senility. Since the FDA prohibits drug manufacturers from disseminating this information to physicians, many health care professionals in the United States are unaware of the manifold uses of this marvelous smart drug.

Hydergine is also good news for cigarette smokers. People who smoke more than 20 cigarettes a day experience a decline of at least 7 percent of the normal blood flow to the brain. This oxygen deprivation causes an increase in the number of free radicals and subsequent damage to brain neurons. Hydergine, a potent free-radical scavenger, may be just what the doctor ordered for tobacco addicts. In addition to neutralizing the toxic molecules that are created when tobacco burns, it may also help lessen the severity of damage to arteries to the brain, a problem caused and aggravated by smoking cigarettes. Of course, it's better not to start smoking in the first place, and it's advisable to quit immediately if you already smoke, but for people who are unwilling or unable to stop smoking, Hydergine (and antioxidant smart nutrients, such as beta-carotene, vitamin E, selenium, L-glutathione, and vitamin C) may provide a large measure of protection against the brain damage that smoking causes.

HOW HYDERGINE WORKS. Hydergine helps increase the delivery of oxygen to the brain (by increasing blood flow) and neutralizes the free radicals that can cause permanent brain damage. Recent research indicates that Hydergine may also stimulate the synthesis of a substance called nerve growth factor that induces the growth of protein filamentous connections between neurons. These connections, called dendrites, facilitate communication throughout the central nervous system and are required for the storage and retrieval of memories. Hydergine also reduces the rate at which lipofuscin accumulates in the brain. Lipofuscin accretion has been implicated as a causative factor in the decline of cognitive functioning as we age.

Since the Sandoz patent on Hydergine has expired, generic brands of dihydrogenated ergot alkaloids or ergoloid mesylates (the chemical names of the brand name Hydergine) are now available from a variety of companies in the United States and Europe. Keep in mind that in the United States, the FDA has approved a dosage of only 3 milligrams per day. The recommended daily dosage for Hydergine in Europe is 9 milligrams—3 milligrams taken three times daily.

Many of the scientific research studies have used dosages closer to or higher than the European dosages, and several have shown that higher dosages of Hydergine produce significantly better results. Some researchers think that it may be best to start with a low dose and work up to larger doses to avoid any uncomfortable side effects, mild as they may be.

PRECAUTIONS: Hydergine is relatively nontoxic. Studies testing four times the FDA-allowed dosage revealed no measurable toxic effects in humans. Hydergine does not cause serious side effects, although there have been occasional reports of mild gastrointestinal discomfort and headaches in a small number of people who use it. These side effects are uncommon and have occurred in individuals who took large doses to start, rather than gradually increased the dosage. Hydergine is essentially nontoxic, even at dosage levels four times higher than those authorized by the FDA. However, people who have chronic or acute psychoses should be advised against it because it could lead to a worsening of the condition. Hydergine is a prescription drug that is currently approved by the FDA only for the treatment of senility; however your physician may legally prescribe it to *prevent* this condition.

Dosage commonly used: 3 mg per day (United States); 9 mg in three divided doses (Europe).

Sources: Hydergine is available as a prescription drug in the United States. Your physician may not yet be familiar with the cognition-enhancing and antiaging effects of Hydergine because the FDA prohibits drug companies from telling physicians about new (FDA unapproved) uses for drugs. There are a wide variety of generic forms of Hydergine, although some generics may not be identical to the original Sandoz formulation (because of a degree of latitude by the FDA in the structural requirements for the generic drug). Some researchers insist that the original Sandoz brand of Hydergine provides superior results than do the generic equivalents.

Centrophenoxine (Lucidril)

Centrophenoxine is a smart drug and a brain antiaging substance based on the molecular formula of the smart nutrient DMAE, commonly found in seafood and nutritional supplements. Like DMAE, centrophenoxine can supply the building blocks for the synthesis of the neurotransmitter acetylcholine. In addition, it can remove lipofuscin deposits in the brain, heart, and skin. Studies have shown that the removal of lipofuscin deposits in the brain is correlated with improved mental functioning, while increased lipofuscin deposits are associated with decreased cognitive abilities.

Centrophenoxine, like DMAE, facilitates nerve transmission across synapses, the tiny spaces between neurons where neurotransmitters are released from one nerve cell to communicate with other nerve cells. Some research indicates that centrophenoxine is as effective as DMAE in neutralizing free radicals. Other research suggests that centrophenoxine is more effective than DMAE in slowing down the accumulation of lipofuscin deposits, at least in experiments on laboratory animals.

PRECAUTIONS: People who are hyperactive, easily excitable, have severe hypertension (high blood pressure), or suffer from or are susceptible to convulsions or involuntary musculoskeletal movements should avoid using centrophenoxine. Nursing mothers should also avoid using this smart drug because it can appear in breast milk. Side effects include insomnia, motion sickness, muscular tremors, hyperexcited states, and even a paradoxical drowsiness. Some instances of depression have also been reported. Centrophenoxine is more likely to cause insomnia if taken late in the day.

Dosage commonly used: 1,000 to 3,000 mg per day.

Sources: Centrophenoxine is not sold in the United States. It can be purchased as an over-the-counter drug in Mexico or by mail order from the sources listed in Appendix I.

Idebenone (Avan)

Idebenone is a smart drug that is structurally related to the smart nutrient coenzyme Q_{10} (CoQ_{10}). CoQ_{10} plays a vital role in the creation of ATP, the primary energy molecule in the body. It has been used in Japan as a treatment for various types of cardiovascular diseases and has been used successfully in the United States as a treatment for gingivitis (inflammatory gum disease).

Several studies have shown that CoQ_{10} can be metabolized in the body in such a way as to create damaging compounds with free radical–like activity, although if the body is supplied with sufficient antioxidant smart nutrients, such as vitamin C, ascorbyl palmitate (fat-soluble vitamin C), beta-carotene, and vitamin E, CoQ_{10} should be able to exert its beneficial effects without causing free-radical damage. Idebenone does not seem to share this problem.

Studies have found that idebenone is relatively nontoxic. No biochemical abnormalities have been noted in people taking idebenone, and no studies I have found report suspicious clinical laboratory values that could be directly related to the use of idebenone.

Dosage commonly used: 100 mg per day.

Sources: Idebenone is not available in the United States and thus must be imported through the mail-order sources listed in Appendix I.

Xanthinol Nicotinate

Xanthinol nicotinate (XN) is structurally related to the smart nutrient vitamin B-3 (niacin): 500 milligrams of XN contain 141.7 milligrams of niacin chemically bonded to a carrier molecule, xanthinol. The advantage to using XN is that it passes through brain-cell membranes and into the cells more easily than does niacin. Once inside the nerve cells, XN stimulates an increase in glucose metabolism, increasing ATP (energy) production. Thus it can increase brain metabolism and energy levels.

XN also behaves as a vasodilator (it opens up blood vessels) and has been shown to reduce blood cholesterol levels. Thus, it can improve the flow of blood to the brain and may be useful in helping prevent stroke and senility.

Research has shown that XN improves reaction times and memory in healthy elderly people when they are given a variety of short-term and long-term memory tests. Other research, testing niacin alone, revealed short-term memory improvements in young and middle-aged individuals.

PRECAUTIONS: XN may cause the same type of skin-flushing reactions as may niacin. Both may also cause heart palpitations, heartburn, vomiting, diarrhea, blurred vision, postural hypotension (dizziness resulting from a drop in blood pressure when standing from a lying or seated position), headache, and liver dysfunction. These side effects are generally transitory and tend to abate once usage is discontinued. Expectant and nursing mothers should avoid the use of XN, as should people with congestive heart failure, peptic ulcer disease, and low blood pressure and those who have suffered recent heart attacks and liver problems.

Dosage commonly used: 1,000–2,000 mg per day in three divided doses taken with meals.

Sources: XN is not available in the United States. It can be purchased in Canada and Europe and by mail order from the sources listed in Appendix I.

A Note About Deprenyl

An FDA-approved drug for the treatment of Parkinson's disease—deprenyl—may actually help boost cognitive functions and may even help delay the onset of Alzheimer's disease. Deprenyl (sold under the name Eldepryl in the United States) has already been shown to extend the life span of laboratory animals. In humans, deprenyl appears to reduce the degradation of important neurotransmitters such as dopamine and norepinephrine. Deprenyl does not appear to be a cure for Alzheimer's disease, but recent studies have shown that it clearly improves the quality of life of Alzheimer's patients and may even slow the progression of the disease. Deprenyl has been shown to reduce the age-related accumulation of lipofuscin and stimulate antioxidant activity in the brain. Interested readers should consult Alastair Dow's book, *Deprenyl: The Anti-Aging Drug* (Hallberg Publishing Corp.; 1993).

9

Eat Smart, Think Smart Recipes

There is no better way to take charge of your mental and physical health than to start by controlling what you put into your body. Smart foods—the ones you've learned about in this book—are easy to find in nearly every supermarket in the world, and they're fun to cook with.

Eating smart may require that you make some slight modifications in the way you ordinarily prepare foods. First and foremost, smart cooking techniques rely on using much less saturated and transfat (found in margarine and certain cooking oils) than do conventional cooking methods. These fats tend to raise blood levels of cholesterol, which can lead to artery closure in the brain. Senility and stroke, two of the most mentally and physically disabling health problems, can be prevented by reducing the amounts of cholesterol and fat in our diets.

Eating smart also means picking smart foods. In *Eat to Win*, I recommended that people choose a variety of colors when shopping for produce. If you remember the acronym ROY GREEN, you'll select red, orange, yellow, and green fruits and vegetables during your next trip to the grocery store. Smart nutrients come packaged, like crayons, in a variety of attractive colors, so when you cover a variety of color bases, you cover a variety of nutritional bases as well:

Red fruits: Tomatoes, strawberries, pink grapefruit, and watermelon, for example, contain the cancer-preventive antioxidant smart nutrients lycopene and beta-carotene; cranberries and raspberries contain anthocyanin, a chemical that keeps the blood from becoming too sticky and clogging arteries. These fruits are also high in vitamin C, another smart antioxidant that helps prevent the formation of cancer-causing chemicals in the gastrointestinal tract. These smart nutrients also protect the brain against free-radical damage, thereby preventing premature brain aging and senility.

Orange-yellow fruits and vegetables: Apricots, cantaloupe, carrots, papaya, mango, sweet potatoes, and yams all contain the antioxidant smart nutrient beta-carotene and hundreds of other carotinoid isomers (similar in molecular structure to beta-carotene). These antioxidants can help prevent various forms of cancer, as well as cardiovascular and cerebrovascular disease (heart attack and stroke).

Green vegetables: Leafy vegetables, including beet and turnip greens, kale, and spinach, contain carotinoids; broccoli and green peppers are rich in vitamin C; and herbs, such as parsley and basil, contain antioxidants called monoterpenes. Even tea (it must be green tea) contains heart disease– and cancer-fighting chemicals called polyols and catechins. Broccoli, cabbage, and kale also contain indoles, which reduce the risk of breast cancer by stimulating the liver to form enzymes that inactivate carcinogens.

About the Recipes

Mamma mia, God bless her, had the patience to spend all day laboring over a hot stove preparing nutritious, home-cooked meals, but with today's microwave mentality, most of us crave the rapid roast and speedy soufflé. We simply can't afford to take the time to make, from scratch, that delicious recipe for Mom's apple pie.

I have three rules for smart cooking at home: simplicity, simplicity, and simplicity! Recipes should always be nutritious and taste delicious, of course, but first and foremost, they should be easy to prepare. That's why I gave Hilarie Porter, MS (who has created custom recipes for my discriminating clients, such as Cher, Don Johnson, Mike Nichols, Martina Navratilova, and Ivan Lendl), the task of creating "quick-smart" recipes that feature smart foods that are rich in antioxidants, vitamins, and minerals, but poor in fat, calories, and cholesterol.

Each recipe has been kitchen tested to ensure ease of preparation and excellent taste. You won't spend a lot of time in the kitchen or shopping for difficult-to-find exotic foods. By combining ordinary supermarket foods in the smart recipes, you'll get the most delicious brain food for the least calories, cholesterol, and fat. Eating smart never tasted so good or was so easy.

A few simple guidelines will help you make the most of these recipes:

Breakfasts. The breakfast recipes contain a smart mix of high-quality protein and complex carbohydrates to supercharge your brain the first thing in the morning. You may use egg substitutes or egg whites in each recipe that calls for eggs (2 egg whites = 1 whole egg).

Salads, Salad Dressings, and Dips. This category emphasizes colors, reflecting the antioxidant smart-nutrient content of the recipes' ingredients. Carrots, broccoli, tomatoes, and cucumbers provide ample free-radical protection, while the dressings and dips minimize the use of fats and oils to help reduce the risk of degenerative diseases, such as stroke and cancer. Try the Quick Caesar Dressing when you want gourmet taste but don't have a lot of time to make dressing from scratch.

Soups. Most of the smart soup recipes contain one of the richest natural sources of smart nutrients, such as choline, that can lift your brain up to maximum mental performance levels. The beans, peas, and lentils in these soups also provide a treasure trove of minerals, such as calcium and magnesium; trace minerals, such as selenium and manganese; and hard-to-get vitamins, such as vitamin E and vitamin B_5. In addition, these legumes will help lower blood cholesterol levels and improve intestinal transit times because they are a rich source of fiber, something most people don't consume in amounts necessary for optimal health.

Breads and Muffins. The Bible refers to bread as the "staff of life." Nutritionists refer to it as a complex-carbohydrate food, rich in fiber, vitamins, and minerals. It all means the same thing: Breads and bread products, such as muffins, supply the body and brain with the most basic energy nutrient—glucose. Your brain needs glucose to think and remember; your muscles need it to move. These bread and muffin recipes will give you all this and *less:* less fat and cholesterol and fewer calories than conventionally made bread products.

Entrées. Seafood and poultry recipes contain a rich supply of smart nutrients, such as DMAE, L-phenylalanine, L-tyrosine, and L-arginine; entrées for vegetarians are based on legumes (beans, peas, and lentils); others include egg whites and whole grains, such as brown rice. All are high in smart nutrients and low in saturated fat and cholesterol for heart-healthy and brain-wise eating.

Desserts. When it's time to wind down from a tough day, these smart desserts give you just what you need—glucose, L-tryptophan, vitamin B_3, and inositol—to help stimulate the release of the neurotransmitter serotonin, in your brain. This smart chemical is vital to falling asleep each night and provides a nondrug means of getting a safe (and deep) night's sleep.

If you have any questions or suggestions regarding these smart recipes, please write to Hilarie Porter at the following address:

Hilarie Porter
PO Box 69-3912
Norland Branch
Miami, FL 33169

Breakfast Dishes

"Bacon" Quiche
Baked Cinnamon Toast
Bananarama Oatmeal
Blueberry Pancakes
Breakfast Pudding
"Dilly" Eggs

"Fried" Muffins
Good Old Scrambled "Eggs"
Italian Omelet
Pasta Omelet
Strawberry Pancakes

Salads, Salad Dressings, and Dips

Basil Dressing
Broccoli-Pasta Salad
Carrot-Pecan Salad
Crab Salad
Cucumber Dressing
Dilled Potato Salad
Green Goddess Dressing
Herb Yogurt Dressing
Italian Bean Salad
Pasta Salad Italiano

Poppy Seed Dressing
Quick Caesar Dressing
Rice Salad
Sesame Seed Dressing
Stuffed Tomatoes
Tomato Dip
Tuna-Dijon Salad
Tuna-Pasta Salad
Vegetable-Herb Dip

Soups

Beany Chili
Cannellini Soup
Creamy Potato Soup
Lentil Soup
Minestrone

Northern Bean Chowder
Pea, Bean, and Lentil Soup
Tomato-Pea Soup
Vegetable Soup

Breads and Muffins

Apple-Nut Bread
Banana Muffins
Banana-Pecan Bread
Bran Muffins
Date Bread

Fruity Oat Muffins
Mexican Corn Bread
Pineapple Muffins
Strawberry Bread

Entrées

Apple Quiche
Balsamic Cod
Black Bean Mexican Pie
Broccoli Casserole
Brown Rice Loaf
Chili Corn Cod
Italian Spinach Bake
Italian-Style Sole
Last-Minute Lasagna

Mexican Snapper
Oven "Fried" Chicken
Spinach-Noodle Casserole
Spinach Frittata
Spinach-Penne Bake
Tarragon-Halibut Steaks
Tuna Stir-Fry
Turkey Chili
Turkey Loaf

Desserts

Apple Cake
Apple Crisp
Banana Cake
Banana-Chip Bars
Brown Frosting
Carrot Cake

Cream Cheese Frosting
Just Because It's Chocolate Cake
Noodle Pudding
Raisin-Pecan Frosting
Spicy Banana Bars

Breakfast Dishes

"Bacon" Quiche

½ cup Bisquick
1 cup fat-free sour cream
½ cup skim milk
½ teaspoon Worcestershire sauce
3 egg whites or egg-substitute
  equivalent

¼ cup finely chopped onion
½ cup chopped green pepper
⅓ cup imitation bacon bits
⅔ cup fat-free Cheddar cheese,
  cut into chunks

1. Preheat the oven to 400 degrees. Spray an 8-inch pie pan with PAM.
2. Place the first 5 ingredients in a large bowl. Mix with an electric mixer.
3. Fold in the rest of the ingredients. Blend.
4. Pour into the prepared pie pan. Bake 20–25 minutes, or until a wooden pick inserted in the middle comes out clean.

SERVES 4

Calories	197	Carbohydrates	11.3 g
Protein	13.6 g	Fat	4.1 g
Sodium	1,284 mg	Cholesterol	1.9 mg

Baked Cinnamon Toast

½ teaspoon cinnamon
3 egg whites
½ cup frozen apple juice
  concentrate (100 percent

natural) or a 4-ounce
can
1 packet Butter Buds
8 thin slices whole wheat bread

1. Preheat the oven to 400 degrees. Spray a 9 × 13-inch baking pan with PAM.
2. Beat the first 4 ingredients together until the Butter Buds are dissolved.
3. Soak the bread slices in the egg-white mixture. Do not leave them in the liquid too long; they may fall apart.
4. Arrange the bread slices in the prepared baking pan. Bake 10 minutes. Turn the slices over and bake them another 10 minutes, or until golden

brown. (Before doing so, you may have to wipe out the baking pan and respray it with PAM to avoid a burned look.

5. Sprinkle the bread slices with Equal, or serve with a light pancake syrup.

SERVES 8

Calories	88	Carbohydrates	17.1 g
Protein	3.9 g	Fat	0.8 g
Sodium	264 mg	Cholesterol	1 mg

Bananarama Oatmeal

¼ cup raisins
2 medium bananas, cut in
  quarters lengthwise and sliced
  ½-inch thick

⅛ teaspoon cinnamon
1½ cups water
1 cup instant oatmeal

1. Place the first 4 ingredients in a saucepan.
2. Bring to a rapid boil. Stir in the oatmeal. Turn off the heat immediately. Stir for 1 minute, leaving the saucepan on the burner.
3. Remove the saucepan from the burner and pour the cereal into 2 bowls. Serve piping hot. Sprinkle with sweetener if desired.

SERVES 2

Calories	361	Carbohydrates	79.4 g
Protein	8.9 g	Fat	3.6 g
Sodium	6.1 mg	Cholesterol	0

Blueberry Pancakes

1 cup whole wheat pastry flour
¼ cup all-purpose flour
2 teaspoons baking powder
¼ teaspoon baking soda

2 tablespoons sugar
1 egg white
¾ cup 100 percent apple
  juice
1 cup fresh blueberries

1. Combine the first 5 ingredients in a large bowl. Blend well. Add the rest of the ingredients. Mix.
2. Spray a nonstick frying pan with PAM. Heat to medium high.
3. Pour the batter into the frying pan, a heaping tablespoon at a time, to make several pancakes.

4. Turn the pancakes when they are bubbly and the bubbles are bursting on the top. Cook until the undersides are golden brown.
5. Place the pancakes on a heated platter. Repeat the cooking process. You may need to wipe out the pan and respray it with PAM to avoid a burned look.
6. Serve with a light pancake syrup.

SERVES 8

Calories	120	Carbohydrates	25.6 g
Protein	3.8 g	Fat	0.3 g
Sodium	33 mg	Cholesterol	0

Breakfast Pudding

1.3-ounce package Jell-O Sugar   *½ cup raisins*
*   Free Cook n' Serve Vanilla*   *¼ teaspoon cinnamon*
*   Pudding & Pie Filling*   *2 cups cooked parboiled brown*
2 cups skim milk   *   rice*

1. Place the skim milk and pudding in a saucepan, stirring until blended. Cook the mixture according to the package directions.
2. When the pudding has thickened, add the raisins, cinnamon, and brown rice. Pour the pudding into 4 small cups.
3. Refrigerate for 5 minutes, or until firm. Serve warm.

SERVES 4

Calories	200	Carbohydrates	42.8 g
Protein	6.9 g	Fat	0.8 g
Sodium	94 mg	Cholesterol	2 mg

"Dilly" Eggs

8 egg whites or egg-substitute   *¼ cup skim milk*
*   equivalent*   *½ teaspoon dried dill weed*
1 packet Butter Buds   *Pepper to taste*
1 cup low-fat cottage cheese

1. Place all the ingredients in a food processor or blender. Mix until smooth.
2. Spray a nonstick frying pan with PAM. Heat to medium high.

3. Pour the mixture into the prepared frying pan. Stirring with a rubber spatula, cook the mixture until it is set.

SERVES 4

Calories	83	Carbohydrates	6.0 g
Protein	12.2 g	Fat	0.8 g
Sodium	558 mg	Cholesterol	4 mg

"Fried" Muffins

4 egg whites
½ cup evaporated skimmed milk
3 tablespoons sugar
½ teaspoon vanilla extract

2 packets Butter Buds
¾ teaspoon dried orange rind
6 whole wheat English muffins,
separated into halves

1. Spray a nonstick frying pan with PAM. Combine the first 6 ingredients in a large bowl. Mix them until the Butter Buds have dissolved.
2. Place the muffins in the mixture, cut side down. Soak 30–60 seconds. Turn the muffins and soak the other sides. Set the muffins aside on a plate until you are ready to cook them.
3. Cook the muffins on medium high, cut side down, until golden brown. Turn and cook the other side until golden brown. Repeat the process for the rest of the muffins. You may have to wipe out the frying pan and respray it with PAM to avoid a burned look.
4. Sprinkle with Equal or serve with a light pancake syrup.

SERVES 6

Calories	203	Carbohydrates	32.2 g
Protein	7.2 g	Fat	4.7 g
Sodium	588 mg	Cholesterol	26 mg

Good Old Scrambled "Eggs"

4 egg whites or egg-substitute
equivalent
1 packet Butter Buds
¼ cup skim milk

Pepper to taste
⅛ teaspoon turmeric (for color),
optional

1. Whisk together all the ingredients until the Butter Buds are dissolved.
2. Spray a nonstick frying pan with PAM.

3. Heat the frying pan to medium high. Pour the egg mixture into the heated pan. Stirring with a rubber spatula, cook until the mixture is set.

SERVES 2

Calories	69	Carbohydrates	8.5 g
Protein	7.3 g	Fat	0.5 g
Sodium	610 mg	Cholesterol	2 mg

Italian Omelet

6 egg whites or egg-substitute equivalent
2 tablespoons grated Parmesan cheese
1 tablespoon snipped fresh parsley

¹/₄ teaspoon Italian seasoning
¹/₈ teaspoon pepper
Pinch of garlic powder
1 cup finely chopped zucchini
³/₄ cup sliced fresh mushrooms
¹/₄ cup finely chopped red onion

1. Preheat oven to 350 degrees. Spray a 9-inch pie pan with PAM.
2. Whisk together the first 6 ingredients in a bowl. Set aside.
3. Spray a nonstick frying pan with PAM. Sauté the zucchini, mushrooms, and onions until tender-crisp. Add a little water if needed.
4. Arrange the vegetables in the prepared pie pan. Whip the egg mixture again and pour it over the vegetables.
5. Bake 20–25 minutes, or until the mixture is set. Cut into wedges.

SERVES 4

Calories	53	Carbohydrates	4.1 g
Protein	6.8 g	Fat	1.1 g
Sodium	122 mg	Cholesterol	2 mg

Pasta Omelet

2 cups plain cooked pasta (day old is fine)
4 large egg whites or egg-substitute equivalent
¹/₄ cup plain low-fat yogurt

¹/₄ cup fat-free cottage cheese
¹/₄ skim milk
¹/₄ cup fat-free Cheddar cheese, shredded
Pepper to taste

1. Preheat the oven to 350 degrees. Spray a 9-inch pie pan with PAM.
2. Spread the cooked pasta evenly in the pan.
3. Place the egg whites, yogurt, cottage cheese, and skim milk in a food

processor or blender. Mix until smooth. Stir in the Cheddar cheese. Pour over the pasta.

4. Bake 25–30 minutes, or until the mixture is set.
5. Let the pan stand for a few minutes. Turn the omelet bottom side up onto a serving platter. Cut it into wedges.

SERVES 4

Calories	204	Carbohydrates	36.5 g
Protein	11.4 g	Fat	0.8 g
Sodium	116 mg	Cholesterol	2 mg

Strawberry Pancakes

1 cup whole wheat pastry flour
¹/₄ cup all-purpose flour
2 teaspoons baking powder
¹/₄ teaspoon baking soda
2 tablespoons sugar

³/₄ cup fresh strawberries,
    mashed with a fork
2 egg whites
1 tablespoon skim milk

1. Combine the first 5 ingredients in a bowl. Blend well. Add the rest of the ingredients. Blend.
2. Spray a nonstick frying pan with PAM. Heat to medium high.
3. Pour the batter into the frying pan, a heaping tablespoon at a time.
4. Turn the pancakes when they are bubbly and the bubbles are bursting on the top. Cook until the undersides are golden brown.
5. Place the pancakes on a heated platter. Repeat the cooking process. You may need to wipe the pan out and respray it with PAM to avoid a burned look.
6. Serve with a light pancake syrup or fresh fruit.

SERVES 8

Calories	88	Carbohydrates	17 g
Protein	3.8 g	Fat	0.25 g
Sodium	39 mg	Cholesterol	0.04 mg

Salads, Salad Dressings, and Dips

Basil Dressing

½ cup low-fat buttermilk
3 tablespoons fat-free
  mayonnaise
1 teaspoon dried basil

1 tablespoon lemon juice
⅛ teaspoon garlic powder
Pinch of pepper

1. Place all the ingredients in a bowl. Mix well.
2. Chill. Pour over a fresh vegetable salad and toss to coat.

MAKES 1 CUP

Calories	8	Carbohydrates	1.4 g
Protein	0.51 g	Fat	0.15 g
Sodium	180 mg	Cholesterol	0.47 mg

Broccoli-Pasta Salad

½ cup fat-free Italian dressing
¾ cup fat-free cottage cheese
1 teaspoon Italian seasoning
1¼ teaspoons dried minced
  garlic
3 tablespoons grated Parmesan
  cheese

½ cup coarsely chopped walnuts
2 cups broccoli flowerets,
  steamed until tender-crisp
4 ounces tricolor pasta twists,
  cooked according to package
  directions

1. Place the first 5 ingredients in a food processor or blender. Mix until smooth.
2. Place the walnuts, broccoli, and pasta in a large bowl. Pour the dressing over the pasta mixture. Toss to coat. Chill.

SERVES 4–6

Calories	141	Carbohydrates	11.9 g
Protein	9.2 g	Fat	7.2 g
Sodium	204 mg	Cholesterol	3.1 mg

Carrot-Pecan Salad

5 cups shredded carrots
½ cup finely chopped pecans
¾ cup raisins

¼ cup orange juice
½ cup fat-free mayonnaise
½ cup plain low-fat yogurt

1. Combine the first 3 ingredients in a large bowl.
2. Place the orange juice, mayonnaise, and yogurt in a food processor or blender. Mix until smooth.
3. Pour the mixture over the carrots, pecans, and raisins. Toss to coat. Chill.

SERVES 6

Calories	206	Carbohydrates	35.5 g
Protein	4 g	Fat	7.2 g
Sodium	101 mg	Cholesterol	1.5 mg

Crab Salad

8 ounces shredded crabmeat,
    cooked or canned
½ cup fat-free mayonnaise
1 cup chopped celery

¼ cup finely chopped green
    onion, including the green part
1 teaspoon lemon juice
Pinch of pepper

1. Combine all the ingredients in a bowl. Mix well.
2. Chill.
3. Serve as a sandwich with whole wheat pita bread or on a bed of lettuce.

SERVES 4

Calories	59	Carbohydrates	1.9 g
Protein	10.1 g	Fat	1.1 g
Sodium	174 mg	Cholesterol	56.7 mg

Cucumber Dressing

¼ cup fat-free mayonnaise
¾ cup plain low-fat yogurt
1½ cups seeded and chopped
    cucumbers

1 teaspoon dried minced garlic
1 tablespoon wine vinegar
Pinch of white pepper

1. Place all the ingredients except ½ cup of the cucumbers in a food processor or blender. Blend until smooth.
2. Stir in the rest of the cucumbers. Chill. Pour over a fresh vegetable salad and toss to coat.

MAKES 3 CUPS

Calories	3	Carbohydrates	0.53 g
Protein	0.2 g	Fat	0.09 g
Sodium	5.3 mg	Cholesterol	0.38 mg

Dilled Potato Salad

5 cups potatoes peeled, cubed, and cooked (6–7 medium potatoes)
1 cup sliced celery
½ cup chopped green onion, including the green part
¾ cup radishes, cut in half and sliced

1 cup fat-free mayonnaise
1 teaspoon prepared mustard
1 tablespoon wine vinegar
⅛ teaspoon garlic powder
⅛ teaspoon pepper
1 teaspoon dried dill weed

1. Place the first 4 ingredients in a large bowl. Toss to mix.
2. Mix the rest of the ingredients in a small bowl. Blend well.
3. Pour over the potato mixture. Toss to coat. Chill.

SERVES 6

Calories	129	Carbohydrates	28.9 g
Protein	3.8 g	Fat	0.19 g
Sodium	58.2 mg	Cholesterol	0

Green Goddess Dressing

½ cup plain low-fat yogurt
½ cup fat-free mayonnaise
2 tablespoons lemon juice
2 tablespoons wine vinegar
¼ cup chopped fresh parsley
¼ cup chopped green onion,

including some of the green part
⅛ teaspoon tarragon
Pinch of white pepper
½ teaspoon anchovy paste
1 teaspoon dried minced garlic

1. Place all the ingredients in a food processor or blender. Mix until smooth. Chill.
2. Pour over a vegetable salad and toss to coat.

MAKES 1 CUP

Calories	31	Carbohydrates	4.1 g
Protein	2 g	Fat	0.92 g
Sodium	293 mg	Cholesterol	4.8 mg

Herb Yogurt Dressing

1 cup plain low-fat yogurt
1/2 cup fat-free mayonnaise
1 teaspoon dried minced garlic
2 tablespoons finely chopped onion

1/2 cup chopped fresh parsley
1/4 cup minced fresh dill
1/4 teaspoon dried tarragon
3 tablespoons balsamic vinegar

1. Place all the ingredients in a food processor or blender. Mix until smooth.
2. Chill. Serve over a fresh vegetable salad and toss to coat.

MAKES 1 1/2 CUPS

Calories	31	Carbohydrates	4.8 g
Protein	1.9 g	Fat	0.7 g
Sodium	36.9 mg	Cholesterol	3.0 mg

Italian Bean Salad

19-ounce can cannellini beans (Italian white beans), drained and rinsed
19-ounce can red kidney beans, drained and rinsed
1 cup chopped red onions
1/2 cup chopped celery

2 tablespoons snipped fresh parsley
1/4 cup lemon juice
1/4 fat-free Italian salad dressing
2 tablespoons Dijon mustard
1/2 teaspoon dried oregano
1/4 teaspoon pepper

1. Place the first 5 ingredients in a large bowl. Mix.
2. Place the rest of the ingredients in a small bowl. Mix well.
3. Pour over the bean mixture and toss to coat. Chill.

SERVES 5

Calories	298	Carbohydrates	55.1 g
Protein	18.2 g	Fat	1.7 g
Sodium	205 mg	Cholesterol	0

Pasta Salad Italiano

3 cups rotelle (pasta twists),
    cooked according to package
    directions
½ cup sliced green olives
½ cup chopped red pepper
½ cup finely chopped red onion

½ cup fat-free mayonnaise
½ cup fat-free Italian salad
    dressing
⅛ teaspoon garlic powder
½ teaspoon basil
⅛ teaspoon pepper

1. Place the first 4 ingredients in a large bowl. Set aside.
2. Place the rest of the ingredients in a small bowl. Mix well. Pour over the
   pasta mixture and toss to coat. Chill.

SERVES 4

Calories	221	Carbohydrates	38.2 g
Protein	6.6 g	Fat	4.7 g
Sodium	883 mg	Cholesterol	0

Poppy Seed Dressing

½ cup chopped onion
¼ cup sugar
1 teaspoon dry mustard
1 teaspoon Tamari soy sauce

⅓ cup oil-free Italian salad
    dressing
⅓ cup balsamic vinegar
1 tablespoon poppy seeds

1. Place all the ingredients in a food processor or blender. Run the motor
   for 10–15 seconds.
2. Chill. Pour over a fresh vegetable salad and toss to coat.

MAKES 1½ CUPS

Calories	27	Carbohydrates	5.8 g
Protein	0.3 g	Fat	0.4 g
Sodium	67 mg	Cholesterol	0

Quick Caesar Dressing

3 large egg whites
1 large garlic clove
4 anchovy filets
1 tablespoon Worcestershire sauce

¼ cup lemon juice
½ teaspoon pepper
⅓ cup grated Parmesan cheese

1. Place the first 6 ingredients in a food processor or blender. Mix until smooth.
2. Add the Parmesan cheese. Mix until blended.
3. Chill. Toss with romaine lettuce.

MAKES ³/₄ CUP

Calories	65	Carbohydrates	2.4 g
Protein	6.7 g	Fat	3.2 g
Sodium	1.3 g	Cholesterol	15 mg

Rice Salad

2 cups cooked brown rice
¹/₂ cup shredded carrots, packed
   solid in a measuring cup
10-ounce package frozen peas,
   thawed and drained
¹/₂ cup plain low-fat yogurt

¹/₂ cup fat-free mayonnaise
1 teaspoon wine vinegar
1 tablespoon Dijon mustard
¹/₈ teaspoon garlic powder
¹/₄ teaspoon pepper
Pinch of curry

1. Place the first 4 ingredients in a large bowl. Mix well.
2. Place the rest of the ingredients in a small bowl. Blend well. Pour over brown-rice mixture. Toss to coat. Chill.

SERVES 4

Calories	170	Carbohydrates	33.3 g
Protein	6.6 g	Fat	1.5 g
Sodium	145.9 mg	Cholesterol	2.3 mg

Sesame Seed Dressing

2 tablespoons toasted sesame
   seeds
¹/₂ cup fat-free Italian salad
   dressing

¹/₂ teaspoon garlic powder
2 tablespoons balsamic vinegar
2 teaspoons Tamari soy sauce

1. Place all the ingredients in a food processor or blender.
2. Mix 2–3 minutes. Chill several hours.
3. Pour over a fresh vegetable salad and toss to coat.

MAKES 1 CUP

Calories	47	Carbohydrates	3.3 g
Protein	1.8 g	Fat	3.4 g
Sodium	318 mg	Cholesterol	0

Stuffed Tomatoes

4 medium-size firm tomatoes
1¼ cup cubed chicken breasts,
  cooked
½ cup fat-free mayonnaise
2 tablespoons chopped green
  onion, including some of the
  green part

½ teaspoon dried dill weed
⅛ teaspoon garlic powder
Pinch of pepper
Pinch of paprika

1. Cut off the tops of the tomatoes. Scoop out the flesh of the tomatoes. Remove the seeds and chop the pulp to equal one cup. Set aside.
2. Place the tomatoes upside down to drain the excess liquid.
3. Place the rest of the ingredients in a bowl. Add the chopped tomato. Mix well.
4. Spoon the mixture into the tomatoes. Sprinkle top with paprika. (If you are not going to serve the tomatoes immediately, do not fill the tomatoes, but refrigerate the filling and the upside-down tomatoes separately until you are ready to serve.)

SERVES 4

Calories	110	Carbohydrates	7.3 g
Protein	16.3 g	Fat	1.9 g
Sodium	50.2 mg	Cholesterol	40.3 mg

Tomato Dip

½ cup fat-free cottage cheese
½ cup plain low-fat yogurt

2 tablespoons dried onion
½ cup chopped, seeded tomato

1. Place the first 3 ingredients in a food processor or blender. Mix until smooth.
2. Place the mixture in a bowl. Stir in the tomato. Chill.
3. Serve with fresh vegetables.

SERVES 12

Calories	19	Carbohydrates	2.5 g
Protein	1.7 g	Fat	0.3 g
Sodium	45 mg	Cholesterol	1 mg

Tuna-Dijon Salad

6½-ounce can solid white tuna,
  packed in spring water
⅓ cup low-fat yogurt
1 tablespoon Dijon mustard
¼ cup finely chopped celery

¼ cup finely chopped red onion
⅛ teaspoon dried dill weed
⅛ teaspoon celery seed
Pepper to taste

1. Place all the ingredients in a bowl. Mix well.
2. Chill. Serve with whole wheat bread or pita.

SERVES 4

Calories	77	Carbohydrates	2.5 g
Protein	14 g	Fat	1 g
Sodium	473 mg	Cholesterol	30.5 mg

Tuna-Pasta Salad

⅓ cup chopped green onion,
  including some of the green
  part
½ cup sliced celery
¼ cup plain low-fat yogurt
¾ cup fat-free mayonnaise
3 tablespoons grated Parmesan
  cheese

2 teaspoons dried parsley
⅛ teaspoon pepper
6½-ounce can solid white tuna,
  packed in spring water,
  drained
8 ounces pasta shells, cooked
  according to the package
  directions

1. Combine the first 8 ingredients in a large bowl. Mix well.
2. Add the pasta shells. Toss to coat. Chill.

SERVES 4

Calories	177	Carbohydrates	20.6 g
Protein	18.2 g	Fat	2 g
Sodium	137.7 mg	Cholesterol	33 mg

Vegetable-Herb Dip

1 cup fat-free cottage cheese
1/4 cup chopped green onion,
   including some of the green
   part

1/2 teaspoon thyme
1/4 teaspoon garlic powder
1/4 teaspoon dill weed
1/4 teaspoon crushed red pepper

1. Place all the ingredients in a food processor or blender. Mix until smooth.
2. Chill.
3. Serve with fresh vegetables or as a potato topper.

SERVES 8

Calories	20	Carbohydrates	1.5 g
Protein	3.4 g	Fat	0.01 g
Sodium	105.2 mg	Cholesterol	1.3 mg

Soups

Beany Chili

1 1/2 cups chopped onions
1/2 cup chopped green pepper
1 tablespoon dried minced garlic
1 tablespoon water
2 8-ounce cans chopped
   tomatoes, undrained

8-ounce can tomato sauce
3 15 1/2-ounce cans pinto beans,
   drained and rinsed
11-ounce can corn, drained
2 1/2 tablespoons chili powder

1. Spray a Dutch oven with PAM. Place the onions, green pepper, garlic, and water in the pot. Sauté until tender-crisp.
2. Add the rest of the ingredients. Bring to a boil. Reduce heat to medium-low. Simmer, uncovered, 40–50 minutes, or until beans are tender. Stir frequently while cooking.

SERVES 10

Calories	214	Carbohydrates	41.3 g
Protein	12.2 g	Fat	1.2 g
Sodium	337 mg	Cholesterol	0

Cannellini Soup

1 cup chopped onions
1½ teaspoons dried minced
    garlic
½ cup sliced celery
28-ounce can chopped tomatoes,
    drained
⅛ teaspoon pepper
19-ounce can cannellini (Italian

white beans), drained and
    rinsed
6 cups defatted chicken broth
1½ cups elbow macaroni
1 packet Butter Buds
2 tablespoons grated Parmesan
    cheese

1. Spray a Dutch oven with PAM. Place the onions, garlic, and celery in the pot. Cook until just tender.
2. Add the tomatoes, pepper, and beans. Cook 2–3 minutes. Add the chicken broth. Bring to a boil. Reduce heat and simmer 5 minutes, uncovered.
3. Add the macaroni. Cook on medium high 8–10 more minutes, or until the macaroni is tender.
4. Stir in the Butter Buds and the Parmesan cheese.

SERVES 12

Calories	158	Carbohydrates	28 g
Protein	9.7 g	Fat	0.9 g
Sodium	561 mg	Cholesterol	1 mg

Creamy Potato Soup

1 cup chopped onions
3 cups skim milk
1 teaspoon Worcestershire sauce
Pinch of white pepper
¼ teaspoon dry mustard
1 packet Butter Buds

Pinch of nutmeg
5 cups potatoes, cooked, cubed,
    and peeled (6–7 medium
    potatoes)
2 tablespoons snipped fresh
    parsley

1. Spray a large Dutch oven with PAM. Place the onions in the pot. Brown on medium high. Add a little water, if necessary, while cooking.
2. Add the rest of the ingredients except the parsley. Mix well.
3. Pour the soup mixture into a food processor or blender, one cup at a time. Turn the motor on and off to blend; the potatoes should be in

small chunks. Return the mixture to the Dutch oven. Repeat the process until all the soup is blended.

4. Heat the soup on medium high; *do not boil.* Add the parsley.

SERVES 5

Calories	267	Carbohydrates	55.3 g
Protein	11.2 g	Fat	0.9 g
Sodium	295 mg	Cholesterol	3 mg

Lentil Soup

³/₄ cup chopped onions
³/₄ cup chopped celery
1 cup sliced carrots
1 teaspoon dried minced garlic
6 cups water
28-ounce can chopped Italian tomatoes, undrained

12-ounce bag brown lentils, rinsed and drained
¹/₂ teaspoon crushed rosemary
¹/₂ teaspoon oregano
¹/₄ teaspoon dried dill weed
¹/₈ teaspoon pepper

1. Spray a Dutch oven with PAM. Place the onion, carrots, and garlic in the pot. Sauté the vegetables until tender-crisp. Add a little of the water if necessary.
2. Add the rest of the ingredients. Bring to a boil. Reduce the heat to medium low and simmer, uncovered, for 40–50 minutes, or until the lentils are tender.

SERVES 10

Calories	151	Carbohydrates	28.1 g
Protein	9.7 g	Fat	0.6 g
Sodium	138 mg	Cholesterol	0

Minestrone

¹/₂ cup chopped onion
¹/₂ teaspoon dried minced garlic
¹/₄ cup sliced carrot
¹/₄ cup sliced celery
3 cups water
32-ounce can peeled whole tomatoes or 2 cups fresh tomatoes, peeled and chopped

15-ounce can low-sodium tomato sauce
15-ounce can pinto beans, drained and rinsed
2 cups ditalini pasta
2 cups sliced zucchini
1 teaspoon Italian seasoning
¹/₄ teaspoon pepper
¹/₄ teaspoon dried dill weed

1. Spray a Dutch oven with PAM.
2. Place the onion, garlic, carrots, and celery in the pot. Sauté on medium-

high heat until the vegetables are tender-crisp. Add a little bit of the water, if necessary.

3. Add the rest of the ingredients. Break up the tomatoes with the back of a wooden spoon while cooking. Simmer, uncovered, 15–20 minutes, or until the pasta is tender.

SERVES 10

Calories	98	Carbohydrates	19.3 g
Protein	4.6 g	Fat	0.8 g
Sodium	441 mg	Cholesterol	0

Northern Bean Chowder

¹/₂ cup chopped onion
¹/₂ cup chopped green pepper
1¹/₂ cups potatoes peeled, cubed, and cooked (1 large potato)
2 cups water

2 15¹/₂-ounce cans Great Northern beans, drained and rinsed
11-ounce can corn, drained
2 packets Butter Buds
¹/₈ teaspoon white pepper

1. Spray a Dutch oven with PAM. Place the onion and green pepper in the pot and sauté until tender. Add a little of the water, if needed, while cooking.
2. Add the potatoes. Mash the potatoes with the back of a wooden spoon, leaving some chunks.
3. Add the rest of the ingredients. Bring to a boil. Reduce the heat to low. Simmer, uncovered, 30–40 minutes, or until the soup thickens.

SERVES 7

Calories	192	Carbohydrates	42.3 g
Protein	10.2 g	Fat	1.5 g
Sodium	712 mg	Cholesterol	2 mg

Pea, Bean, and Lentil Soup

2 cups assorted peas, beans, and lentils (rinsed and placed in a Dutch oven, covered with water, and soaked overnight)
9 cups water
2 cups chopped onions
28-ounce can chopped tomatoes, undrained
2 cloves garlic, minced

3 tablespoons imitation bacon bits
1 teaspoon chili powder
2 teaspoons Italian seasoning
1 teaspoon salt
1 bay leaf
1 cup small fusilli pasta

1. Drain excess water off the beans. Place all the ingredients except the pasta in a Dutch oven. Bring to a boil.
2. Reduce the heat to medium. Simmer, uncovered, 3–4 hours, or until the beans are tender.
3. When the beans are tender, add the pasta and cook 10–12 more minutes.

SERVES 11

Calories	289	Carbohydrates	50.8 g
Protein	16.7 g	Fat	2.6 g
Sodium	787 mg	Cholesterol	0

Tomato-Pea Soup

1 cup chopped onions
12-ounce package dry split peas
4 cups V-8 vegetable juice
3 cups defatted chicken broth

³/₄ teaspoon garlic powder
¹/₄ teaspoon pepper
1 packet Butter Buds
1 bay leaf

1. Place all the ingredients in a large saucepan. Bring to a boil.
2. Cover. Reduce the heat. Simmer 60 minutes, or until the peas are tender. Stir occasionally.
3. Place the soup in 1–2 cup batches in a food processor or blender. Puree. Return to the saucepan and reheat.

SERVES 6

Calories	265	Carbohydrates	48.4 g
Protein	17.9 g	Fat	0.6 g
Sodium	629 mg	Cholesterol	0

Vegetable Soup

¹/₂ cup sliced carrots
¹/₂ cup sliced celery
¹/₂ cup chopped onions
10-ounce package frozen peas
14¹/₂-ounce can defatted chicken broth
1¹/₂ cups water
1 teaspoon dried parsley
1 teaspoon Tamari soy sauce
¹/₈ teaspoon pepper

³/₄ teaspoon garlic powder
28-ounce can chopped Italian tomatoes, drained
8-ounce can tomato sauce
16-ounce can red kidney beans, drained
Grated Parmesan cheese to sprinkle on individual servings (1 to 2 teaspoons)

1. Spray a Dutch oven with PAM. Place the carrots, celery, and onions in the pot. Cook on medium-high heat until tender. Add a little of the water, if needed, while cooking.
2. Add the rest of the ingredients. Bring to a boil. Reduce the heat and simmer, uncovered, 15–20 minutes.

SERVES 8

Calories	130	Carbohydrates	24 g
Protein	8 g	Fat	0.7 g
Sodium	560 mg	Cholesterol	0

Bread and Muffins

Apple-Nut Bread

2 cups whole wheat pastry flour
³/₄ cup chopped walnuts
1 teaspoon baking soda
1 teaspoon baking powder
¹/₂ cup sugar
2 cups Red Delicious apples,

peeled, cored, and finely
chopped
2 egg whites
1¹/₂ cups 100 percent apple juice
1 teaspoon vanilla

1. Preheat the oven to 350 degrees. Spray a 5 × 9-inch loaf pan with PAM.
2. Place the first 5 ingredients in a large bowl. Blend. Add the apples.
3. Whisk together the rest of the ingredients in a small bowl. Pour into the apple mixture. Blend well.
4. Pour into the prepared loaf pan. Bake 50–60 minutes, or until a wooden pick inserted in the middle of the loaf comes out clean.

SERVES 10

Calories	180	Carbohydrates	32.7 g
Protein	2.9 g	Fat	4.3 g
Sodium	78 mg	Cholesterol	0

Banana Muffins

1¼ cups whole wheat pastry
   flour
1 cup rolled oats
¼ cup bran
1½ teaspoons baking powder
½ teaspoon baking soda
½ cup sugar
1 cup dried banana chips

¼ cup Red Delicious apples,
   peeled, cored, and shredded,
   and packed solid in measuring
   cup
1 cup ripe banana, mashed (2–3
   medium bananas)
1 cup skim milk
2 egg whites
1 teaspoon vanilla

1. Preheat the oven to 350 degrees. Spray a 12-cup muffin pan with PAM.
2. Combine the first 7 ingredients in a large bowl. Add the shredded apples and mashed bananas. Blend well.
3. Whisk together the rest of the ingredients in a separate bowl. Pour into the flour mixture. Blend well.
4. Spoon the batter into the prepared muffin pan until each cup is about ¾ full.
5. Bake 20–25 minutes, or until a wooden pick inserted in the middle of a muffin comes out clean.

MAKES 12 MUFFINS

Calories	129	Carbohydrates	27.3 g
Protein	3.4 g	Fat	0.7 g
Sodium	53 mg	Cholesterol	0

Banana-Pecan Bread

1 cup sugar
1½ cups mashed ripe bananas
½ cup soft butter-flavored light
   margarine
¼ cup low-fat buttermilk
3 egg whites
1½ cups all-purpose flour

½ cup whole wheat flour
1 teaspoon baking soda
½ teaspoon salt
2 teaspoons dried grated orange
   rind
½ cup chopped pecans

1. Preheat the oven to 350 degrees. Spray a 5 × 9-inch loaf pan with PAM.
2. Place the first 10 ingredients in a large bowl. Mix with an electric mixer until smooth. Fold in the pecans. Pour into the prepared loaf pan.

3. Bake 50–60 minutes, or until a wooden pick inserted in the middle comes out clean.

SERVES 10

Calories	250	Carbohydrates	50 g
Protein	4.7 g	Fat	4.6 g
Sodium	202.6 mg	Cholesterol	0.09 mg

Bran Muffins

*1¼ cups whole wheat pastry
    flour
¾ cup bran
¾ cup rolled oats
1 cup sugar
1½ teaspoons baking powder
½ teaspoon baking soda
¼ teaspoon cinnamon
½ teaspoon dried orange rind*

*¾ cup raisins
½ cup Red Delicious apples,
    peeled, cored, and shredded,
    and packed solid in measuring
    cup
1 cup low-fat buttermilk
2 egg whites
1 teaspoon vanilla*

1. Preheat the oven to 350 degrees. Spray a 12-cup muffin pan with PAM.
2. Combine the first 10 ingredients in a large bowl. Mix well.
3. Whisk together the rest of the ingredients in a small bowl. Pour into the flour mixture. Blend well.
4. Spoon the batter into the prepared muffin pan until each cup is about ¾ full.
5. Bake 20–25 minutes, or until a wooden pick inserted in the middle of a muffin comes out clean.

MAKES 12 MUFFINS

Calories	174	Carbohydrates	39.8 g
Protein	3 g	Fat	0.7 g
Sodium	52 mg	Cholesterol	0

Date Bread

*1 cup pitted chopped dates
1 cup raisins
1½ cups boiling water
2 cups whole wheat pastry flour
1 tablespoon sugar
1 teaspoon baking soda
1 teaspoon baking powder
1 teaspoon dried orange rind*

*1 packet Butter Buds
½ cup chopped walnuts
2 egg whites
1 teaspoon vanilla
½ cup Red Delicious apples,
    peeled, cored, and shredded,
    and packed solid in measuring
    cup*

1. Preheat the oven to 350 degrees. Spray a 5 × 9-inch loaf pan with PAM.
2. Place the dates and raisins in a bowl. Pour boiling water over them. Mix. Set aside to cool.
3. Combine the next 7 ingredients in a large bowl. Mix well.
4. Add the date mixture to the flour. Mix well. Add the egg whites and vanilla. Blend.
5. Pour into the prepared loaf pan.
6. Bake 40–50 minutes, or until a wooden pick inserted in the middle of the loaf comes out clean.

SERVES 10

Calories	187	Carbohydrates	38.7 g
Protein	3.2 g	Fat	3 g
Sodium	163 mg	Cholesterol	0

Fruity Oat Muffins

1½ cups rolled oats
1¼ cups whole wheat pastry
flour
¾ cup sugar
3 tablespoons bran
1½ teaspoons baking powder
¾ teaspoon baking soda
½ teaspoon cinnamon
⅓ cup raisins

⅓ cup dried banana chips, broken into small pieces
¼ cup dried pineapple, cut into small pieces
½ cup Red Delicious apples, peeled, cored, and shredded, and packed solid in measuring cup
¼ cup chopped pecans
1 cup skim milk
2 egg whites

1. Preheat the oven to 400 degrees. Spray a 12-cup muffin pan with PAM.
2. Place the first 12 ingredients in a large bowl. Mix well.
3. Add the skim milk and egg whites. Mix until the batter is moistened.
4. Spoon the batter into the prepared muffin pan until each cup is about ¾ full. Bake 15–20 minutes, or until a wooden pick inserted in the middle of a muffin comes out clean.

MAKES 12 MUFFINS

Calories	190	Carbohydrates	37.8 g
Protein	4.3 g	Fat	2.9 g
Sodium	72 mg	Cholesterol	0

Mexican Corn Bread

1 cup yellow cornmeal
1 cup all-purpose flour
2 teaspoons sugar
1 tablespoon baking powder
1/2 teaspoon salt
2 tablespoons dried onion
1 cup skim milk
2 egg whites

1/4 cup soft butter-flavored light
   margarine
15-ounce can corn, drained
4-ounce can chopped green
   chilies
1/2 cup fat-free Cheddar cheese,
   shredded

1. Preheat the oven to 425 degrees. Spray an 8 × 8-inch baking dish with PAM.
2. Place the first 6 ingredients in a large bowl. Mix well.
3. Place the skim milk, egg whites, and margarine in another bowl. Whisk together.
4. Add to the dry mixture and blend. Fold in the chilies and the Cheddar cheese.
5. Pour into the prepared baking pan. Bake 25–30 minutes, or until a wooden pick inserted in the middle of the corn bread comes out clean.

SERVES 8–10

Calories	95	Carbohydrates	18.3 g
Protein	3.5 g	Fat	1.3 g
Sodium	150.8 mg	Cholesterol	33.3 mg

Pineapple Muffins

1 1/2 cups whole wheat pastry
   flour
3/4 cup rolled oats
1/4 cup bran
1 1/2 teaspoon baking powder
1/2 teaspoon baking soda
1/4 teaspoon nutmeg
1/4 cup sugar
3/4 cup chopped fresh pineapple

(or drained unsweetened
   canned pineapple chunks)
1/4 cup chopped walnuts
1/4 cup Red Delicious apples,
   peeled, cored, and shredded,
   and packed solid in measuring
   cup
1 cup skim milk
2 egg whites
1/2 teaspoon vanilla

1. Preheat the oven to 350 degrees. Spray a 12-cup muffin pan with PAM.
2. Combine the first 10 ingredients in a large bowl. Mix well.

3. Whisk together the rest of the ingredients in another bowl. Pour into the flour mixture. Blend well.
4. Spoon the batter into the prepared muffin pan until each cup is ³/₄ full.
5. Bake 20–25 minutes, or until a wooden pick inserted in the middle of a muffin comes out clean.

MAKES 12 MUFFINS

Calories	142	Carbohydrates	27.9 g
Protein	3.8 g	Fat	2 g
Sodium	55 mg	Cholesterol	0

Strawberry Bread

1¹/₂ cups all-purpose flour
1 cup sugar
1 teaspoon baking powder
¹/₂ teaspoon salt
1 teaspoon vanilla
¹/₂ cup butter-flavored light margarine

3 egg whites
¹/₄ cup skim milk
16-ounce bag frozen whole unsweetened strawberries, defrosted and mashed

1. Preheat the oven to 350 degrees. Spray a 5 × 9-inch loaf pan with PAM.
2. Place the first 4 ingredients in a large bowl. Mix.
3. Mix the rest of the ingredients in another bowl with an electric mixer. Gradually add to the dry mixture. Blend until smooth. Fold in the strawberries.
4. Pour into the prepared loaf pan. Bake 1 hour, or until a wooden pick inserted in the middle of the loaf comes out clean.

SERVES 10

Calories	154	Carbohydrates	35 g
Protein	3.2 g	Fat	0.5 g
Sodium	152.7 mg	Cholesterol	0.12 mg

Entrées

Apple Quiche

*½ pound turkey sausage (about 4
  sausages)*
½ cup chopped onions
¼ teaspoon thyme
*1½ cups tart apples, peeled,
  cored, and cubed*
1 tablespoon lemon juice

1 tablespoon sugar
*1 cup fat-free Cheddar cheese,
  shredded*
*4 egg whites or egg-substitute
  equivalent*
1½ cups skim milk

1. Preheat the oven to 350 degrees. Spray a 9-inch pie pan with PAM.
2. Brown the turkey sausages and onions in a nonstick frying pan. Add the
   thyme. Cook until the sausages are browned and the onions are clear.
   Drain the excess fat. Slice sausages and set aside.
3. Place the apples, lemon juice, and sugar in a large bowl. Add the
   sausage mixture and the cheese. Mix well.
4. Beat together the eggs and milk. Pour over the sausage mixture. Blend.
5. Pour into the prepared pie pan. Bake 45–50 minutes, or until the
   mixture is set.

SERVES 8

Calories	122	Carbohydrates	10.2 g
Protein	7.8 g	Fat	5.7 g
Sodium	234 mg	Cholesterol	15.9 mg

Balsamic Cod

2 pounds cod fillets (four fillets)
*2–3 tablespoons balsamic
  vinegar*

2–3 teaspoons garlic powder
Pepper to taste

1. Preheat the broiler.
2. Place the fillets on a broiling pan that has been covered with aluminum
   foil.

3. Brush the fillets with vinegar.
4. Sprinkle the fillets evenly with garlic powder and pepper.
5. Broil 7–10 minutes, or until the fillets flake when pricked with a fork.

SERVES 4

Calories	389	Carbohydrates	1 g
Protein	64.8 g	Fat	12.1 g
Sodium	250 mg	Cholesterol	183.8 mg

Black Bean Mexican Pie

1 cup chopped onions
1/2 cup chopped green pepper
2 teaspoons chili pepper
1/2 teaspoon garlic powder
1/8 teaspoon salt
16-ounce can black beans,
*   drained*

1 1/2 cups brown rice
3/4 cup skim milk
3 egg whites, lightly beaten
1 cup fat-free Cheddar cheese,
*   shredded*

1. Preheat the oven to 350 degrees. Spray a 9-inch pie pan with PAM.
2. Place all the ingredients in a large bowl. Mix.
3. Pour into the prepared pie pan. Bake 25–30 minutes, or until the center is set.

SERVES 6

Calories	167	Carbohydrates	30.6 g
Protein	10 g	Fat	0.9 g
Sodium	97.8 mg	Cholesterol	0.6 mg

Broccoli Casserole

2 10-ounce packages frozen
*   chopped broccoli, defrosted*
*   and well drained*
5 egg whites or egg-substitute
*   equivalent, well beaten*
2 cups fat-free cottage cheese
1/2 cup fat-free sour cream

1/2 cup sliced mushrooms
1/4 cup chopped green onions
1/8 teaspoon salt
1/8 teaspoon pepper
2 tablespoons grated Parmesan
*   cheese*

1. Preheat the oven to 350 degrees. Spray a 9 × 13-inch baking pan with PAM.

2. Place all the ingredients except the Parmesan cheese in a large bowl. Mix well. Pour into the baking pan. Sprinkle the top with Parmesan cheese.
3. Bake 40–45 minutes, or until golden.

SERVES 8

Calories	72	Carbohydrates	7.3 g
Protein	11.1 g	Fat	0.25 g
Sodium	284 mg	Cholesterol	2.5 mg

Brown Rice Loaf

2 cups cooked brown rice
1 cup shredded carrots
1/4 cup chopped onion
1 cup fat-free Cheddar cheese, shredded

3 egg whites, lightly beaten
1/2 cup shelled sunflower seeds
1/8 teaspoon pepper
1/4 teaspoon dill weed

1. Preheat the oven to 350 degrees. Spray a 5 × 9-inch loaf pan with PAM.
2. Place all the ingredients in a large bowl. Mix well.
3. Pour into the prepared loaf pan. Press lightly into the pan to form a loaf.
4. Bake for 45–50 minutes, or until set and the sides are golden.

SERVES 4

Calories	285	Carbohydrates	31.1 g
Protein	11.8 g	Fat	14.1 g
Sodium	70.1 mg	Cholesterol	0

Chili Corn Cod

1 pound cod fillets, 1/2–1-inch thick
2 teaspoons butter-flavored light margarine
2 teaspoons chili powder
1 1/2 teaspoons dried onion

10-ounce package frozen corn, defrosted and drained
1/4 cup chopped red pepper
1/4 cup chopped green pepper
1 teaspoon Tamari soy sauce
1/4 cup water

1. Preheat the broiler. Spray a broiling pan with PAM.
2. Place the fillets on the prepared broiling pan. Broil 4 minutes. Turn and broil 4–5 minutes on the other sides, or until the fillets are flaky when touched with a fork.

3. In the meantime, melt the margarine. Add the water, chili powder, corn, onion, red pepper, green pepper, and Tamari and stir. Cook 2–3 minutes on high heat, reduce the heat, and simmer uncovered until the fillets are done.
4. Cut the fillets into four equal portions. Spoon the corn mixture over them. Serve immediately.

SERVES 4

Calories	154	Carbohydrates	15.3 g
Protein	22.4 g	Fat	1.1 g
Sodium	169.4 mg	Cholesterol	56.7 mg

Italian Spinach Bake

15-ounce can tomato sauce
2 tablespoons grated Parmesan
  cheese
1 teaspoon basil
1 teaspoon oregano
2 cloves garlic, minced
10-ounce package frozen

chopped spinach, defrosted
  and drained
1 medium onion, thinly sliced
  and rings separated
2 medium tomatoes, thinly sliced
4 ounces fat-free mozzarella,
  shredded

1. Preheat the oven to 350 degrees.
2. Combine the first 5 ingredients in a bowl. Set aside.
3. Spray an 8 × 8-inch baking pan with PAM. Layer the vegetables in the baking pan in the following order: tomatoes, onions, spinach; then spread with tomato sauce. Repeat the layers and spread the tomato sauce on the top layer. Sprinkle the top with the mozzarella.
4. Bake covered 20–25 minutes. Remove the cover and bake 10–15 minutes more, or until the cheese has melted and is golden.

SERVES 4

Calories	130	Carbohydrates	16.9 g
Protein	14.6 g	Fat	1.4 g
Sodium	841.5 mg	Cholesterol	6.9 mg

Italian-Style Sole

1 pound sole fillets, 1/4–1/2-inch
  thick (4 fillets)
2 egg whites
1 tablespoon lemon juice

1/8 teaspoon pepper
1/2 teaspoon garlic powder
1/2 cup Italian bread crumbs
1/4 cup Parmesan cheese

1. Preheat the broiler.
2. Spray a broiling pan with PAM.
3. Place the egg whites and lemon juice in a small bowl. Beat together with a whisk.
4. Place the rest of the ingredients in another bowl. Mix.
5. Dip the fillets in the egg mixture and coat well. Then dip them in the bread-crumb mixture and coat them lightly.
6. Place the fillets on the broiling pan. Broil 2–3 minutes on one side. Turn the fillets and broil them 2–3 minutes on the other sides until golden and flaky when touched with a fork.

SERVES 4

Calories	185	Carbohydrates	11.3 g
Protein	21.3 g	Fat	5.5 g
Sodium	292.8 mg	Cholesterol	49.8 mg

Last-Minute Lasagna

1 pound ground turkey
½ cup chopped onion
1 teaspoon dried minced garlic
½ teaspoon crushed red pepper
26-ounce jar marinara sauce
16-ounce can tomato sauce
½ teaspoon oregano
½ teaspoon basil
2 tablespoons grated Parmesan cheese

2 cups fat-free cottage cheese
1 cup fat-free mozzarella, shredded
12 ounces lasagna noodles, uncooked
1 cup sliced mushrooms
1 cup chopped red peppers
1 cup chopped yellow peppers

1. Preheat oven to 375 degrees. Spray a 9 × 13-inch baking pan with PAM.
2. Place the turkey, onion, and garlic in a Dutch oven with a little bit of water. Cook on medium-high heat until the turkey is browned and the liquid has evaporated.
3. Add the marinara sauce, tomato sauce, oregano, basil, and crushed red pepper. Simmer 10–15 minutes.
4. Spread a little sauce on the bottom of the prepared baking pan. Place part of the *uncooked* noodles on the bottom of the baking pan. Spread half the cottage cheese over the noodles evenly. Spread half the sauce over the cottage cheese. Arrange the vegetables on top of the sauce. Sprinkle the Parmesan cheese over the vegetables. Top with the

remaining noodles. Place the rest of the sauce on top of the noodles. Sprinkle the top with the mozzarella.
8. Cover with aluminum foil.
9. Bake 45–50 minutes. Remove the foil and bake 10–15 more minutes, or until the cheese is golden and bubbly.

SERVES 10

Calories	305	Carbohydrates	36.2 g
Protein	25.9 g	Fat	5.9 g
Sodium	852 mg	Cholesterol	39.7 mg

Mexican Snapper

1 tablespoon butter-flavored light margarine
2 cups chopped tomatoes
2 tablespoons lime juice
2 tablespoons chopped green chilies

¼ teaspoon garlic powder
⅛ teaspoon pepper
Pinch of pepper
1 pound snapper fillets
¼ cup chopped green onion, including the green part

1. Preheat the broiler. Spray a broiling pan with PAM.
2. Place the first 7 ingredients in a saucepan. Bring just to a boil. Reduce the heat and simmer 10–15 minutes, or until the snapper is done.
3. In the meantime, place the fillets on the broiling pan. Broil 3–4 minutes. Turn the fillets and broil 3–4 minutes more on the other sides, or until they are flaky when touched with a fork.
4. Cut the fillets into four equal portions. Spoon the tomato mixture over them. Sprinkle with the green onion.

SERVES 4

Calories	259	Carbohydrates	14 g
Protein	34.4 g	Fat	7.3 g
Sodium	746.1 mg	Cholesterol	91 mg

Oven "Fried" Chicken

¼ cup flour
¼ cup whole wheat flour
½ teaspoon garlic powder
¼ teaspoon pepper
⅛ teaspoon marjoram
½ teaspoon salt

2 egg whites
½ cup low-fat buttermilk
4½ cups cornflakes, crushed
4 tablespoons sesame seeds
2–3 pound broiler-fryer chicken, cut up, with the skin removed

1. Preheat the oven to 375 degrees. Line a large baking pan with aluminum foil.
2. Place the first 6 ingredients in a bowl. Mix well. Beat together the egg whites and the buttermilk in another bowl.
3. Place the cornflakes and sesame seeds in another bowl. Mix.
4. Dip the chicken, one piece at a time, into the flour mixture, then into the buttermilk, and then into the cornflakes-and-sesame-seed mixture, coating evenly.
5. Place the chicken pieces in the baking pan.
6. Bake 50–60 minutes, or until the chicken is golden.

SERVES 6–8

Calories	685	Carbohydrates	86.4 g
Protein	57.2 g	Fat	11.3 g
Sodium	785 mg	Cholesterol	148.2 mg

Spinach-Noodle Casserole

8 ounces no-yolk noodles, cooked according to the package directions

2 10-ounce packages frozen chopped spinach, defrosted and drained

1 tablespoon soft butter-flavored light margarine

1 cup chopped onions

5 egg whites or egg-substitute equivalent, well beaten

1 cup fat-free sour cream

½ cup fat-free mozzarella, shredded

½ cup fat-free Cheddar cheese, shredded

⅛ teaspoon pepper

1. Preheat the oven to 350 degrees. Spray a 3–4 quart casserole with PAM.
2. Place the noodles in a large bowl. Add the rest of the ingredients. Toss to mix.
3. Pour the mixture into the prepared casserole. Bake covered for 30 minutes. Remove the cover and bake 15 more minutes.

SERVES 8

Calories	56	Carbohydrates	8.1 g
Protein	6.1 g	Fat	0.4 g
Sodium	95.2 mg	Cholesterol	0.9 mg

Spinach Frittata

½ pound turkey sausage
2 cups chopped onions
1 teaspoon dried garlic
½ cup sliced mushrooms
8 egg whites or egg-substitute
   equivalent
½ cup grated Parmesan cheese

½ teaspoon basil
½ teaspoon marjoram
⅛ teaspoon pepper
10-ounce package frozen
   chopped spinach, defrosted
   and well drained
½ cup fat-free mozzarella

1. Preheat the oven to 350 degrees. Spray a 9-inch deep-dish pie pan with PAM.
2. Brown the turkey sausage, onions, and garlic in a nonstick frying pan. Add the mushrooms and cook until just tender. Drain excess fat. Slice sausage.
3. Mix the eggs, Parmesan cheese, basil, marjoram, and pepper. Whisk together until blended.
4. Fold in the spinach and turkey mixture. Pour into the prepared pie pan.
5. Add shredded mozzarella. Mix well.
6. Bake 25–30 minutes or until the eggs are set.

SERVES 6

Calories	194	Carbohydrates	8.8 g
Protein	25.1 g	Fat	7.4 g
Sodium	279 mg	Cholesterol	54.9 mg

Spinach-Penne Bake

2 10-ounce packages frozen
   chopped spinach, thawed and
   drained
1 pound penne noodles, cooked
   according to the package
   directions
2 cups fat-free cottage cheese
2 15½-ounce jars marinara
   sauce

4 egg whites, lightly beaten
⅓ cup grated Parmesan cheese
⅓ cup chopped fresh parsley
½ teaspoon pepper
1 teaspoon Italian seasoning
⅔ cup fat-free Cheddar cheese,
   shredded
⅓ cup fat-free mozzarella,
   shredded

1. Preheat the oven to 350 degrees. Spray a 9 × 13-inch baking pan with PAM.
2. Combine the first 9 ingredients and ⅓ cup of the Cheddar cheese in a large bowl. Mix well.

3. Pour into the prepared baking pan.
4. Sprinkle the top evenly with the remaining ⅓ cup Cheddar cheese and the mozzarella. Cover the pan with aluminum foil.
5. Bake 25–30 minutes. Remove the foil and bake another 10–15 minutes, or until the cheese is bubbly and golden.

SERVES 10

Calories	216	Carbohydrates	37.4 g
Protein	15.8 g	Fat	1.9 g
Sodium	445 mg	Cholesterol	4.8 mg

Tarragon-Halibut Steaks

¼ cup vegetable oil
2 tablespoons lemon juice
1 teaspoon tarragon

⅛ teaspoon pepper
2 teaspoon Tamari soy sauce
1 pound halibut steaks

1. Preheat the broiler. Spray the broiling pan with PAM.
2. Place the first 5 ingredients in a small bowl. Whisk together to mix. Spoon half the mixture on the fish. Broil 5–6 minutes on one side. Turn the fish and spoon the rest of the mixture on the other sides. Broil 5–6 more minutes, or until the fish is flaky when touched with a fork. Cut into 4 equal portions.

SERVES 4

Calories	322	Carbohydrates	0.8 g
Protein	28.9 g	Fat	21.9 g
Sodium	305 mg	Cholesterol	68.1 mg

Tuna Stir-Fry

2 tablespoons butter-flavored
light margarine
2 tablespoons lemon juice
1 tablespoon Tamari soy sauce
2 tablespoons water
1 teaspoon dried minced garlic
¼ cup chopped celery
¼ cup finely chopped fresh
parsley

2 cups cooked brown rice
6½-ounce can solid white tuna,
packed in spring water
½ cup chopped green onions
⅛ teaspoon pepper
1 tablespoon grated Parmesan
cheese

1. Spray a nonstick frying pan with PAM. Cook the first 4 ingredients at medium-high heat. Add the celery and the parsley. Cook until the celery is just tender.
2. Add the brown rice, stirring constantly to coat it with the mixture. Blend in the tuna, onions, pepper, and Parmesan cheese. Cook until heated through.
3. Serve immediately.

SERVES 4

Calories	170	Carbohydrates	21.3 g
Protein	16.4 g	Fat	1.8 g
Sodium	678 mg	Cholesterol	30.8 mg

Turkey Chili

1 tablespoon butter-flavored light margarine
2 cups chopped onions
1 cup chopped green pepper
½ pound ground turkey
½ pound turkey sausage, chopped
3 teaspoons minced garlic
2 28-ounce cans whole tomatoes, with juice
3 tablespoons chopped green chilies

2 teaspoons–2 tablespoons chili powder
⅛ teaspoon pepper
30-ounce can pinto beans, drained and rinsed
15-ounce can kidney beans, drained and rinsed
3 tablespoons imitation bacon bits
½ teaspoon paprika
½ teaspoon garlic powder
⅛ teaspoon allspice

1. Place the first 6 ingredients in a large Dutch oven. Cook at medium heat until the turkey is browned.
2. Add the rest of the ingredients. Simmer 45 minutes to 1 hour, stirring frequently with a wooden spoon. Mash the tomatoes with the spoon while cooking.

SERVES 10

Calories	314	Carbohydrates	39.2 g
Protein	22.1 g	Fat	8.8 g
Sodium	890 mg	Cholesterol	26.9 mg

Turkey Loaf

Loaf

1 pound ground turkey
½ cup chopped green pepper
2 egg whites
½ cup skim milk
½ cup quick-cooking rolled oats
1 tablespoon dried minced onion

1 teaspoon dried parsley flakes
⅛ teaspoon Tamari soy sauce
⅛ teaspoon pepper
¼ cup catsup
½ teaspoon mustard
½ teaspoon Worcestershire sauce

Sauce

¼ cup catsup
½ teaspoon mustard

½ teaspoon Worcestershire

1. Preheat the oven to 350 degrees. Spray a 5 × 9-inch loaf pan with PAM.
2. Place all the ingredients for the loaf in a large bowl. Mix well. Pour into the prepared loaf pan. Spread evenly and press lightly into a loaf shape. Set aside.
3. Mix all the ingredients for the sauce in a small bowl. Spread evenly on top of the loaf.
4. Bake 35–40 minutes. Spoon off any excess fat.
5. Bake 5–10 more minutes or until the meat is no longer pink in the middle.

SERVES 6

Calories	176	Carbohydrates	13.7 g
Protein	18.8 g	Fat	0.6 g
Sodium	332.9 mg	Cholesterol	49.9 mg

Desserts

Apple Cake

2 cups flour
1 cup whole wheat flour
1¹/₂ cups sugar
¹/₂ cup raw sugar
1 teaspoon baking soda
¹/₂ teaspoon salt
¹/₂ teaspoon cinnamon
1 cup soft butter-flavored light
   margarine

4 egg whites, lightly beaten
2 teaspoons vanilla
¹/₂ cup chopped pecans
¹/₂ cup raisins
4 cups Rome apples, peeled,
   cored, and chopped

1. Preheat the oven to 350 degrees. Spray a 9 × 13-inch baking pan with PAM.
2. Place all the ingredients in a large bowl. Mix well.
3. Pour into the prepared baking pan. Bake 45–50 minutes, or until a wooden pick inserted in the middle comes out clean.

SERVES 10

Calories	322	Carbohydrates	69.5 g
Protein	4.4 g	Fat	4.3 g
Sodium	179 mg	Cholesterol	0

Apple Crisp

6 medium Rome apples, peeled,
   cored, and sliced
2 tablespoons lemon juice
1 tablespoon water
1 teaspoon sugar
³/₄ cup brown sugar

¹/₂ cup whole wheat flour
¹/₂ cup rolled oats
¹/₂ teaspoon cinnamon
¹/₂ cup soft butter-flavored light
   margarine

1. Preheat the oven to 375 degrees.
2. Arrange apples in an 8 × 8-inch baking pan. Sprinkle with the lemon juice, water, and one teaspoon of sugar.

3. Combine the rest of the ingredients in a small bowl. Mix with a fork until the mixture is crumbly.
4. Sprinkle the mixture evenly over the apples.
5. Bake 40–45 minutes, or until the apples are tender.

SERVES 6

Calories	328	Carbohydrates	81.5 g
Protein	2.4 g	Fat	1.4 g
Sodium	72.2 mg	Cholesterol	0

Banana Cake

1¼ cups flour
1 cup whole wheat flour
1 cup sugar
¼ raw sugar
2½ teaspoons baking powder
½ teaspoon baking soda
¼ teaspoon salt

1½ cups ripe bananas, mashed
   well
½ cup soft butter-flavored light
   margarine
3 egg whites
1 teaspoon vanilla extract

1. Preheat the oven to 350 degrees. Spray 2 8-inch cake pans with PAM. Flour thc sides and bottom of the cake pans.
2. Place all the ingredients in a large bowl. Blend with an electric mixer until smooth.
3. Pour the batter into the prepared cake pans. Bake 25–30 minutes, or until a toothpick inserted in the middle comes out clean.
4. Cool 10 minutes. Remove from the pans and cool completely.
5. When cooled, frost with Raisin-Pecan Frosting (see p. 162).

SERVES 12

Calories	204	Carbohydrates	47.5 g
Protein	3.9 g	Fat	0.8 g
Sodium	93.7 mg	Cholesterol	0

Banana-Chip Bars

2 cups all-purpose flour
¾ cup whole wheat flour
1¼ cups sugar
1¼ cups ripe bananas, mashed well
¾ cup soft butter-flavored light
   margarine

4 egg whites
1¼ teaspoons baking powder
1¼ teaspoons baking soda
6-ounce package chocolate chips

1. Preheat the oven to 350 degrees. Spray a 9 × 13-inch baking pan with PAM.
2. Place the first 8 ingredients in a large bowl. Blend with an electric mixer until smooth. Fold in the chocolate chips.
3. Bake 25–30 minutes, or until a wooden pick inserted in the middle comes out clean.

SERVES 12

Calories	308	Carbohydrates	54.1 g
Protein	13.1 g	Fat	5.2 g
Sodium	112 mg	Cholesterol	0

Brown Frosting

¼ cup butter-flavored light margarine

2 cups powdered sugar
3–4 tablespoons skim milk

1. Melt the margarine in a saucepan over low heat, stirring constantly until it turns light brown.
2. Remove from the heat and gradually beat in the powdered sugar with an electric mixer. Beat in the skim milk gradually until the mixture is smooth and can be spread. Add more of the milk if frosting becomes dry.

MAKES 1 CUP

Calories	101	Carbohydrates	25.5 g
Protein	0.13 g	Fat	0.6 g
Sodium	4.5 mg	Cholesterol	0.08 mg

Carrot Cake

1¼ cups flour
1¼ cups whole wheat pastry flour
1½ cups sugar
½ cup raw sugar
2 teaspoons baking soda
½ teaspoon cinnamon
¼ teaspoon salt
1 teaspoon dried orange peel

2 cups shredded carrots
½ cup chopped pecans
½ cup raisins
8-ounce can crushed pineapple, drained
6 egg whites
1¼ cups soft butter-flavored light margarine

1. Preheat the oven to 350 degrees. Spray 2 8-inch cake pans with PAM.
2. Combine the first 8 ingredients in a large bowl. Add the carrots, pecans, raisins, and pineapple. Blend.
3. Beat the egg whites and margarine together with an electric mixer until smooth. Add to the dry mixture. Mix well with a wooden spoon.
4. Pour into the prepared cake pans. Bake 45–50 minutes, or until a toothpick inserted in the middle comes out clean.
5. Cool 10 minutes before removing the layers from the pans. Frost with Cream Cheese Frosting (below).

SERVES 12

Calories	304	Carbohydrates	63.6 g
Protein	5.5 g	Fat	4.4 g
Sodium	95.9 mg	Cholesterol	0

Cream Cheese Frosting

*8-ounce package light cream
  cheese*

*2 teaspoons vanilla extract
3 cups powdered sugar*

1. Place the cream cheese in a bowl. Gradually add the sugar and vanilla, beating with an electric mixer.
2. Mix until smooth.

MAKES 4 CUPS

Calories	188	Carbohydrates	39.6 g
Protein	2 g	Fat	3.3 g
Sodium	107.1 mg	Cholesterol	10 mg

Just Because It's Chocolate Cake

*8¼-ounce package devil's food
  cake mix*
*4½-ounce package chocolate
  fudge pudding mix*
1 cup fat-free sour cream

*½ cup soft butter-flavored light
  margarine*
½ cup warm water
4 egg whites
2 cups semisweet chocolate chips

1. Preheat the oven to 350 degrees. Spray a 9-inch Bundt cake pan with PAM.
2. Place the cake mix and pudding mix in large bowl. Mix. Add the sour

cream, margarine, water, and egg whites. Blend with an electric mixer until smooth.

3. Fold in the chocolate chips. Pour the batter into the prepared Bundt pan. Bake 40–50 minutes, or until a wooden pick inserted in the middle of the cake comes out clean.

SERVES 12

Calories	176	Carbohydrates	22.3 g
Protein	3.1 g	Fat	8.7 g
Sodium	92.5 mg	Cholesterol	0.2 mg

Noodle Pudding

8-ounce package no-yolk wide noodles, cooked according to the package directions
2 cups fat-free cottage cheese
1 cup fat-free sour cream
8-ounce can crushed pineapple (undrained)

½ cup raisins
2 tablespoons soft butter-flavored light margarine
½ cup sugar
4 egg whites or egg-substitute equivalent
1 teaspoon vanilla extract

1. Preheat the oven to 350 degrees. Spray a 2–3 quart casserole with PAM.
2. Place the first 5 ingredients in a large bowl. Place the rest of the ingredients in a blender or food processor. Mix until smooth.
3. Pour over the noodle mixture. Blend.
4. Pour into the prepared casserole. Bake 1 hour.

SERVES 10

Calories	128	Carbohydrates	24.7 g
Protein	7.5 g	Fat	0.3 g
Sodium	193.7 mg	Cholesterol	2.2 mg

Raisin-Pecan Frosting

8-ounce package light cream cheese
2½ cups powdered sugar

½ cup raisins
½ cup chopped pecans

1. Place the cream cheese in a bowl. Gradually beat in the powdered sugar with an electric mixer.

2. Mix until smooth. Stir in the raisins and the pecans.

MAKES 4 CUPS

Calories	213	Carbohydrates	38.9 g
Protein	2.6 g	Fat	6.6 g
Sodium	107.8 mg	Cholesterol	10 mg

Spicy Banana Bars

2 cups mashed ripe bananas	2 cups flour
²/₃ cup brown sugar	1 teaspoon baking soda
¹/₄ cup butter-flavored light margarine	¹/₂ teaspoon baking powder
	2 teaspoons pumpkin pie spice
3 egg whites	¹/₂ cup raisins

1. Preheat the oven to 350 degrees. Spray a 9 × 13-inch baking pan with PAM.
2. Place the first 8 ingredients in a large bowl. Mix with an electric beater until smooth.
3. Fold in the raisins. Pour into the prepared baking pan. Bake 25–30 minutes, or until a wooden pick inserted in the middle comes out clean.
4. Frost with Brown Frosting (see page 160), or serve plain.

SERVES 12

Calories	197	Carbohydrates	46.5 g
Protein	3.7 g	Fat	0.5 g
Sodium	103 mg	Cholesterol	0

Glossary

Acetylcholine: a neurotransmitter involved primarily in memory, sensory input, and muscular movement. Acetylcholine is synthesized from the smart nutrient choline. See also **Lecithin** and **DMAE**.

Alzheimer's disease: a disease that causes severe memory impairment; striking personality changes; and loss of speech, judgment, and intellectual ability. The most common cause of dementia, Alzheimer's disease generally reveals itself after the age of fifty. Currently, the prognosis for the disease is grim. The disease inexorably takes from a few months to five years to obliterate the victim's intellectual function. Some researchers speculate that the lifelong use of antioxidant smart nutrients may help prevent senility, in general, and Alzheimer's disease, in particular.

Amino acid: a molecule that contains an ammonialike compound (amine group), coupled with an organic acid (carboxyl group) that forms the building blocks of all proteins. The human body requires twenty-two specific amino acids. Twelve of them can by synthesized by the body (called nonessential amino acids), whereas ten must be obtained from foods (essential amino acids).

Anabolic substance: a drug, hormone, or nutrient that causes growth. The amino acids L-arginine and L-ornithine, certain synthetic and natural steroids, the herb ephedra (ephedrine), the mineral complex chromium picolinate, and human growth hormone are a few examples of anabolics.

Antioxidant: a natural or synthetic chemical or a nutrient that inactivates the damaging portion (active site) of free radicals. Antioxidants also help neutralize chemicals that cause the formation of free radicals. Vitamins A, B_1, B_5, B_6, C, E, and beta-carotene; the minerals selenium and zinc; coenzyme Q_{10}; uric acid; and three enzymes in the body (superoxide dismutase, catalase, and glutathione peroxidase) are all antioxidants. By neutralizing free radicals, antioxidants prevent damage to cell membranes and genetic material, such as DNA.

Ascorbic acid: the chemical name for vitamin C (other common forms of vitamin C are calcium ascorbate and sodium ascorbate).

Ascorbyl palmitate: a fat-soluble form of vitamin C that exhibits powerful antioxidant properties. Ascorbyl palmitate is a nutritional supplement and does not occur naturally in foods.

ATP (adenosine triphosphate): the universal energy molecule in nature. ATP is created in the mitochondria (energy center of each cell) using energy derived from foods that are consumed. When ATP is split by enzymes, energy is released for various cellular functions and muscular contractions.

BCAA: the acronym for branched-chain amino acid. The BCAAs—leucine, isoleucine, and valine—are used by muscle tissue for energy during exercise. The BCAAs, most notably leucine, can be converted to sugar via the liver during times of physical activity.

BCKA: an acronym for branched-chain keto acid. The BCKAs are formed when BCAAs are deaminated (have an ammonia molecule removed). BCKAs can be used as a nonnitrogen source of energy by the body. BCKA supplements reduce the body's requirement for protein because they can pick up an ammonia molecule and transform into BCAAs.

Beta-carotene (pro-vitamin A): a yellowish pigment found in plants, such as squash, carrots, and pumpkin. The beta isomer of carotene pigment is the most biologically active of pro-vitamin A, so called because in mammals, a liver enzyme splits one molecule of beta-carotene in half, forming two molecules of active vitamin A. Beta-carotene is a powerful antioxidant; it neutralizes a damaging type of activated oxygen called singlet oxygen.

Bioflavonoids: a group of compounds, including hesperidin and rutin, that work synergistically with vitamin C to maintain healthy blood vessels and a healthy immune system. Bioflavonoids are commonly found in many fruits, vegetables, wine, and tea.

Biotin: a nutrient that acts as a coenzyme in metabolic reactions (carboxylations and decarboxylations) involving fats, proteins, and carbohydrates. Biotin deficiency can lead to depression.

Boron: a trace mineral required for bone and muscle growth. Recent research suggests that boron may help prevent muscle loss due to aging and also help prevent osteoporosis by stimulating bone mineralization.

Calcium ascorbate: the calcium salt of vitamin C that is less acidic than vitamin C.

Catabolism: the metabolic process of degradation. Catabolism occurs during periods of exercise, stress, and protein/calorie deficiency, and results in loss of muscle tissue, triglyceride (stored fat), and glycogen (stored carbohydrate).

Catalase: an antioxidant enzyme that catalyzes the breakdown of hydrogen peroxide in cells. Catalase is found in all aerobic organisms that require oxygen or can survive in its presence.

Catecholamines: a group of brain neurotransmitters (chemicals that communicate messages between nerves), including norepinephrine and dopamine. All catecholamines are synthesized from the two amino acids L-phenylalanine and L-tyrosine.

Conversion of Phenylalanine and Tyrosine to Catecholamines

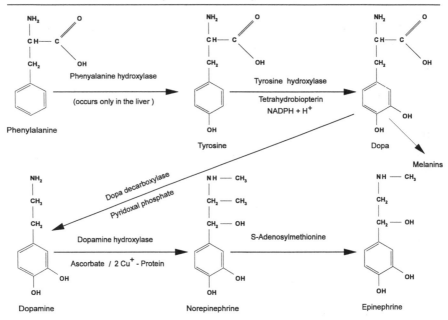

Central nervous system: the brain, spinal cord, glands, and nerves encased within the membranes surrounding the brain and spinal cord.

Centrophenoxine: the generic name for the smart drug Lucidril. The active molecule of centrophenoxine is the smart nutrient DMAE.

Cerebrospinal fluid: a water-based liquid cushion that protects the brain and spinal cord from physical trauma. The fluid contains a large concentration of vitamin C.

Cholesterol: a sterol manufactured in the liver and other cells and found only in animal protein and fats and oils (one exception: spirulina, a blue-green algae, contains cholesterol). The body uses cholesterol to synthesize hormones and cell membranes. High levels of plasma cholesterol (called LDL) are associated with an increased risk of cardiovascular disease. Oxidized cholesterol is suspected as the primary culprit in damage to arteries.

Choline: associated with the B-vitamin family. Choline is converted to the neurotransmitter, acetylcholine in the brain. It can serve as a smart nutrient, boosting memory and mental energy.

Cholinergic: the parts of the nervous system that use acetylcholine as a neurotransmitter. Acetylcholine is released at the synaptic junction (a connecting space between nerves, nerves and muscles, nerves and organs). Acetylcholine is involved in memory, sexual activity, and long-term planning.

Chromium: an element required for the metabolism of carbohydrates. Chromium helps the hormone insulin clear the blood of glucose and move it into cells.

Chromium picolinate: a special form of chromium, developed by a scientist at the U.S. Department of Agriculture that is several times more effective than chromium. Chromium picolinate seems to aid in the loss of fat and muscle building in people who use it during periods of intense exercise and caloric control.

Coenzyme Q$_{10}$: a substance synthesized by the body responsible for the synthesis of adenosine triphosphate (ATP), the universal energy molecule. Research suggests that coenzyme Q$_{10}$ acts as a fat-soluble free-radical neutralizer and helps regulate the electrical conduction system of the heart.

Corpus callosum: a bundle of nerve fibers that connects the two hemispheres of the brain.

Cysteine: a sulfur-containing amino acid with antioxidant properties.

d-Alpha tocopherol: natural vitamin E.

Deanol: the generic name for DMAE.

Degenerative disease: the gradual deterioration of a biological system resulting from damage by free radicals.

Dendrites: the fine network of branches that extend from the body of a nerve cell, receiving impulses and carrying them into the center of the cell.

Dihydrogenated ergot alkaloids: one of the generic names for the prescription drug Hydergine (see Ergoloid mesylates).

DMAE (dimethylaminoethanol): a nutrient that provides raw materials for the synthesis of choline and the neurotransmitter acetylcholine. DMAE stimulates the incorporation of choline into cell membrane lipids and acts as a reservoir for choline during times of choline deficiency.

DNA (deoxyribonucleic acid): the genetic blueprint that resides in the nucleus of every cell of every living organism. Many researchers believe that free-radical damage to the DNA is directly involved in aging and cancer.

Dopamine: a neurotransmitter that is critical to fine motor coordination; immune function; motivation; insulin regulation; physical energy; thinking; short-term memory; emotions, such as sexual desire; and maintaining balance in the autonomic nervous system.

Dopaminergic: the parts of the nervous system that use dopamine as a neurotransmitter.

Enzymes: complex proteins that are capable of inducing chemical changes in other substances without being changed themselves.

Ergoloid mesylates: one of the generic names for the prescription drug Hydergine.

Free radical: a highly chemically reactive atom, molecule, or molecular fragment with a free or unpaired electron. Free radicals are produced in many different ways such as: normal metabolic processes, ultraviolet radiation from the sun, nuclear radiation, and the breakdown of spoiled fats in the body. Free radicals have been implicated in aging, cancer, cardiovascular disease, and other kinds of damage to the body. See also **Antioxidant.**

Free-radical reaction: the cascade of chemical reactions that occurs when a free radical reacts with another molecule to gain an electron. The molecule that loses an electron to the free radical then becomes a free radical, repeating the process until the energy of the free radical is spent or the reaction is stopped by an antioxidant. In biological systems this cascade can damage important molecules like DNA.

Free-radical theory of aging: the theory developed by Dr. Denham Harman at the University of Nebraska that postulates that damage by free radicals is the root cause of the damage to biological systems that we know as aging and chronic degenerative disease.

GABA (gamma aminobutyric acid): an amino acid that acts as an inhibitory neurotransmitter.

Generic drug: a drug that is sold under its technical name rather than under a single company's brand or trade name. A generic drug is marketed when the time period on the patent held by the original manufacturer has expired. By law, a generic drug must contain the same ingredients and be at the same strength as the brand-name drug for which it is substituted. Generic drugs are usually much less expensive than are their brand-name equivalents.

Ginkgo biloba: an herbal extract from the ginkgo tree that stimulates cerebral circulation and improves mental functioning.

Glutathione peroxidase: a sulfur-containing enzyme that possesses powerful antioxidant properties. Each molecule of glutathione peroxidase contains four molecules of selenium.

Growth hormone: a hormone secreted by the pituitary gland. It stimulates growth and repair of the body, as well as the activities of the immune system. With age, its release diminishes.

Hormone: a chemical messenger, such as growth hormone, testosterone, or insulin.

Hypoxia: a condition of lowered oxygen levels in the blood. It promotes free-radical activity in the body.

Inhibitory neurotransmitter: a neurotransmitter that decreases the electrochemical activity of neurons. GABA and serotonin are inhibitory neurotransmitters.

Inositol: a sugar-related smart nutrient that promotes sleep when used with vitamin B_3 (niacinamide) and GABA (gamma aminobutyric acid, an inhibitory neurotransmitter).

L-arginine: an amino acid that stimulates the release of two growth-related hormones, insulin and human growth hormone. L-arginine is also used by the body to help dispose of ammonia that accumulates during protein metabolism.

L-carnitine: a molecule synthesized in the body that shuttles fatty acids into and out of the mitochondria where it is burned for energy. L-carnitine also stimulates the synthesis of the universal energy molecule, adenosine triphosphate (ATP).

L-carnosine: a free radical–neutralizing molecule that acts as a storage site for the amino acid L-histidine. The eye lens contains a high concentration of L-carnosine, which protects it against free-radical damage.

L-cysteine: an antioxidant sulfur-containing amino acid.

Lecithin: a compound called phosphatidyl choline. It is a source of choline that, in turn, is a precursor of the neurotransmitter acetylcholine in brain chemistry. Lecithin is part of the structural material for every cell in the human body.

L-histidine: an amino acid that is converted into histamine, an irritating substance that causes inflammation of skin, eyes, nose, and throat, especially during colds and allergies.

Lipofuscin: the brown waste material deposited in skin and nerve cells that is commonly called age spots. It is made of free radical–damaged proteins and fats.

Liver spots: deposits of lipofuscin in skin.

L-phenylalanine: an amino acid that is a precursor for the neurotransmitter norepinephrine.

L-taurine: an amino acid that helps protect the eye from free-radical damage, helps regulate the electrical conduction system in the heart, and acts as a regulatory/inhibitory neurotransmitter in the brain.

L-tryptophan: an amino acid used in the synthesis of the neurotransmitter serotonin. L-tryptophan stimulates the release of growth hormone from the pituitary gland, helps relieve pain, and produces a relaxed, sleepy state when consumed with carbohydrate-rich/protein-poor foods. The body can convert small amounts of L-tryptophan into vitamin B_3 (niacinamide).

L-tyrosine: an amino acid that is a precursor of the neurotransmitters dopamine and norepinephrine, found in high concentrations in the brain.

Manganese: a cofactor in many enzyme-mediated reactions. It is essential for the production of the antioxidant enzyme SOD.

Methionine: a sulfur-containing amino acid with antioxidant properties.

Methyl xanthines: a class of compounds that can stimulate mental alertness, fight fatigue and depression, and enhance thermogenesis (fat-burning). Common methyl xanthines are caffeine, theobromine, and theophylline.

Mitochondria: the "power plants" inside cells where oxygen and nutrients are metabolized to water, carbon dioxide, and energy.

Nerve: a cell that carries information to and from the central nervous system.

Nerve growth factor (NGF): a naturally occurring hormone that stimulates the growth of neurites.

Neurites: the tiny projections growing from each nerve cell that carry information from cell to cell. A nerve cell may have over 100,000 neurites growing out of it, each connected to another nerve cell.

Neurochemical: a chemical that naturally occurs in the nervous system and plays a part in its functioning.

Neuron: a nerve cell; the structural and functional unit of the nervous system.

Neurotransmitter: one of the many chemicals that carries impulses between nerve cells.

Nitric oxide: a short-lived neurotransmitter (half-life: 6 to 10 seconds) that controls blood flow and is involved in a myriad of bodily functions involving the immune and cardiovascular systems. Nitric oxide was recently discovered to play a key role in penile erection.

Nootropic: a new class of drugs providing desirable qualities of cerebral stimulation and enhancement without the negative side effects of ordinary psychoactive drugs. The word was coined by Dr. C. Giurgea from the Greek *noos = mind; tropein = toward.*

Norepinephrine: an excitatory neurotransmitter involved in alertness, concentration, aggression, and motivation. It is made in the brain from the amino acids L-phenylalanine and L-tyrosine.

Oxidation: a type of chemical reaction in which an electron is removed from the compound being oxidized. Removing an electron creates a free radical (a compound lacking an electron or with an unpaired electron). Oxygen is the most common oxidizing compound.

Parkinson's disease: a chronic disease of the central nervous system caused by lowered levels of the inhibitory neurotransmitter dopamine. Symptoms include muscular tremors and weakness.

Phosphatidyl choline: a phospholipid (fat) that the body can use as a precursor to make choline. Phosphatidyl choline is also effective in lowering serum cholesterol.

Piracetam: a drug that exhibits characteristics of enhancing intelligence, memory, and teaming, as well as slowing down and preventing aspects of brain aging.

Pituitary gland: a gland at the base of the brain. The pituitary secretes several different hormones involved in key metabolic processes.

Placebo: an inert compound usually given to a portion of the subjects in a scientific experiment to distinguish the psychological effects of the experiment from the physiological effects of the drug being tested.

Potassium: a mineral responsible for transmitting electrical impulses. It is highly active in the tissues of the brain and nervous system.

Precursor: a chemical that can be converted by the body into another.

Receptors: sites on the outside of cells where particular messenger molecules, such as hormones, can attach. This attachment to the receptor site causes corresponding changes inside the cell.

RNA (ribonucleic acid): a nucleic acid that controls the protein synthesis in all cells; RNA is required for memory. Animal studies suggest that RNA supplements may improve memory.

Selenium: an important trace mineral with antioxidant properties. Selenium and antioxidant enzymes containing selenium have shown strong anticancer properties.

Senility: the aging-related loss of mental faculties.

Serotonin: an inhibitory neurotransmitter required for sleep.

Singlet oxygen free radical: a single molecule of oxygen that has gained an extra electron. This is a highly reactive state; the singlet oxygen free radical is one of the most destructive free radicals known. Internally, it is a toxic by-product of many metabolic reactions. Smoking is the largest single producer of the singlet oxygen free radical.

Stroke: a rupture in a blood vessel in the brain, often with disastrous effects, depending on where the rupture occurs.

Superoxide dismutase (SOD): an antioxidant enzyme containing zinc and copper or manganese. Its main function is to scavenge and neutral-ize the superoxide free radical.

Synapse: the gap between nerve cells. Chemicals called neurotransmit-ters are the substances that allow nerves to communicate with each other across the synaptic gaps.

Synergy: the action of two or more compounds combined such that their effects are greater than the sum of their individual effects; many of the compounds are said to have positive synergy.

Toxic: poisonous. Everything, including water and oxygen, is toxic in sufficiently high doses.

Unsaturated fats: fats that contain double bonds between some of their carbon atoms. These double-bond positions are vulnerable to attack by oxygen and free radicals.

Vitamin A: one of the fat-soluble vitamins and an important antioxidant. Also called retinol, it is the form of vitamin A that is found in animals. It is essential to growth, healthy skin and epithelial tissue, and the preven-tion of night blindness.

Vitamin B_1 (thiamin): a member of the B complex of vitamins that is essential to the health of brain and nerve tissue. It is also involved in the chemical reactions that cause the release of acetylcholine in the brain.

Vitamin B_2 (riboflavin): a member of the B complex of vitamins that functions as an antioxidant cofactor, taking part in metabolic reactions involving proteins, fats, and carbohydrates.

Vitamin B_3 (niacin): a member of the B complex of vitamins, a defi-ciency of which produces memory failure. Niacin occurs in two forms, nicotinic acid and niacinamide. Both forms are used in smart-nutrient formulas. Niaccin causes skin flushing, burning, stomach acidity, and other side effects that can be harmful to individuals with certain medical conditions. Niacinamide does not cause these side effects.

Vitamin B_5 (pantothenic acid): a member of the B complex of vitamins that acts as an antioxidant. It is also required for the conversion of choline to acetylcholine.

Vitamin B_6 (pyridoxine): a member of the B complex of vitamins that acts as an antioxidant. It is also required for the conversion of amino acids into neurotransmitters in the brain; for example, the conversion of phenylalanine to norepinephrine requires vitamin B_6.

Vitamin B_{12} (cobalamin): a member of the B complex of vitamins that is a particularly important coenzyme in the brain and nerve tissues. It is necessary for the synthesis of DNA, enhances the action of vitamin C and several amino acids, and is required for building the walls of brain cells.

Vitamin C: one of the most important antioxidant nutrients. Also called ascorbic acid, it is essential in building strong, healthy tissue, especially capillary walls.

Vitamin C pump: a biological protective mechanism that steps up the concentration of vitamin C in the spinal fluid and in the brain 100 times greater than the concentration of vitamin C in the circulating blood and body fluids.

Vitamin E: a fat-soluble vitamin that is chemically known as d-alpha-tocopherol. It is one of the main antioxidant nutrients and promotes fertility and prevents abortion.

Zinc: a mineral that is found in substantial concentrations in the brain. It is a necessary factor in over twenty different enzymatic reactions and is essential for the production of the antioxidant enzyme SOD. It also helps prevent the accumulation of lead, which is toxic to the brain.

Sources of Products

The companies listed here can supply smart drugs and/or smart nutrients from national or international sources. Most companies will send a catalog of their products and information on ordering, and some offer free newsletters. These listings are provided for information purposes only.

If you know of additional sources of products, please write to me at the address below, so I can check them out for possible inclusion in future editions of this book:

PO Box 69-3912
Norland Branch
Miami, FL 33169

Smart Drugs from Overseas

You can write to these mail-order smart-drug suppliers for product information. At the present time, the FDA permits the importation of a three-month personal supply of smart drugs (and unapproved AIDS medications).

Baxamed Switzerland Medical Center
Realpstrasse 83
CH-4054 Basel, Switzerland
Fax: 061-301-38-72

Sells a variety of nootropics.

Big-Ben Export Co. (Tudor Trading Co.)
PO Box 146, Mill Hill
London NW7 3DL, England

Sells a variety of nootropics and accepts Visa and Mastercard.

B. Mougios & Co., O.E.
Pittakou 23 T.K.
54645, Thessaloniki, Greece

Sells most of the nootropics at reasonable prices.

Discovery Experimental and Development, Inc.
29949 S.R. 54 West
Wesley Chapel, FL 33534
Telephone (in Mexico): 01-1-5266-304464

Sells inexpensive nootropics manufactured in Mexico.

Note: you can purchase nootropic drugs at the *farmacias* (pharmacies) in Mexico without a prescription and can legally import a personal three-month supply under current FDA regulations.

InHome Health Services
Box 3112
CH-2800 Delemont, Switzerland

Sells nootropics and other drugs.

Interlab
BCM Box 5890
London WC1N 3XX, England

Sells nootropics and other drugs.

Kerwin Whitnah, c/o Fountain Research
PO Box 250
Lower Lake, CA 95457
Telephone: 800-659-1915

Sells a variety of nootropics.

Longevity Plus
U Dubu 27
147 00 Prague 4-Branik, Czech Republic

Sells nootropics.

Masters Marketing Co., Ltd.
Masters House—No. 1, Marlborough Hill
Harrow, Middlesex, HA1 1TW England
Fax: 081-427-1994

Handles a vast range of products, but does not have a catalog. The company will send price quotations on products for which customers fax or write their requests.

Pharmaceuticals International
416 West San Ysidro Boulevard, Suite 37
San Ysidro, CA 92073
Telephone: 800-365-3698

Offers a large variety of other products by written request.

Qwilleran
PO Box 1210
Birmingham B10 9QA, England

Sells most of the nootropics and some AIDS drugs at reasonable prices.

World Health Services
PO Box 20
CH-2822 Courroux, Switzerland

Sells a number of FDA-unapproved European pharmaceuticals.

Consumer alert: On January 29, 1992, the FDA issued an import alert against the following companies: **Interpharm, Inc.** (Bahamas); **Inhome Health Services** (Switzerland); **Northham Medication Service International Pharmacy** (Bahamas); **International Products** (Germany); **Azteca Trio Internacional, S.A. de C.V.** (Mexico); and **Interlab** (England). The FDA has instructed U.S. Customs to detain *all shipments* from these six companies. This import alert may be temporary, so please check before ordering.

Mail-Order Companies That Sell Smart Nutrients

Age Reduction Supplements
8900 Winnetka Avenue, Suite 23
Northridge, CA 91324
Telephone: 800-748-6166
Fax: 818-407-8500

JM Pharmacal
251-B East Hacienda Avenue
Campbell, CA 95008
Telephone: 800-538-4545

This company specializes in selling bulk amino-acid powders at reasonable rates. It will also custom-blend amino-acid mixes of your choice.

Life Services Supplements, Inc.
3535 Route 66
Neptune, NJ 07753
Telephone: 800-542-3230 or 908-922-0009
Fax: 908-922-5329

Distributes products formulated by well-known nutritional scientist, Durk Pearson and Sandy Shaw, two of the first scientists to popularize the general use of smart nutrients, and sells a variety of rationally designed brain formulas and energy-enhancement products.

NutriGuard Research
PO Box 865-A
Encinitas, CA 92023
Telephone: 800-433-2402 or 619-942-3223

Responsible Health, Inc.
3535 East Coast Highway, Suite 231-C
Corona Del Mar, CA 92625
Telephone: 714-720-9110

Smart Products
870 Market Street, Suite 1262-SD
San Francisco, CA 94102
Telephone: 800-858-6520 or 415-989-2500

Offers a free newsletter and sells health-related videos and books in addition to nutritional supplements.

Smart Nutrient Brands in Health Food Stores

Source Naturals
PO Box 2118
Santa Cruz, CA 95063
Telephone: 408-438-6851

Sells Body/Mind supplements, formulated specifically for cognitive enhancement, as well as a variety of nutritional supplements.

Twin Laboratories, Inc.
2120 Smithtown Avenue
Ronkonkoma, NY 11779
Telephone: 800-645-5626 or 516-467-3140

I have known the Blechman family (the owners) for more than twelve years and have helped design a line of nutritional supplement formulas (Endurance brand) for Twin Laboratories. Twin Laboratories manufactures a complete line of nutritional products in capsules, powders, and liquids. Its products are available in most health food and vitamin stores and, in my opinion, are some of the most innovative and highest-quality supplements available on the market today. The company will send a product-information catalog on request.

Additional Smart Drug and Nutrient Sources

Bronson Pharmaceuticals
4526 Rinetti Lane
La Canada, CA 91011
Telephone: 818-790-2646

Sells bulk quantities of vitamins and other products by mail order only. Write or telephone for mailing envelopes.

Emerson Ecologics, Inc.
436 Great Road
Acton, MA 01720
Telephone: 800-654-4432

Distributes a number of nutritional supplements, including a line of herbal formulations manufactured by Murdock Pharmaceuticals.

The Life Extension Foundation
PO Box 229120
Hollywood, FL 33022
Telephone: 1 800-841-LIFE (24-hour toll-free); if you call Monday
  through Friday from 9:00 A.M. to 5:30 P.M., Eastern Standard
  Time, you'll talk to someone who can answer questions about
  products. At other times, you can leave a recorded message.
  Other telephone numbers: in the Hollywood, Florida, area: 305-
  966-4886; in Canada: 800-826-2114

Sells a comprehensive line of nutritional supplements, as well as life-
extension books. It also publishes a monthly newsletter (not free) and has a
toll-free hotline (see above) to answer questions about the products it sells.

Metagenics, Inc.
23180 Del Lago
Laguna Hills, CA 92653
Telephone: 800-692-9400; in California: 800-833-9536

Carries a comprehensive line of nutritional supplements, including many
of those discussed in this book.

Omnitrition International, Inc.
1620 Rafe Street, Suite 108
Carrollton, TX 75006
Telephone: 800-446-1025 or 214-702-7600

PWA Health Group
31 West 26th Street, 4th floor
New York, NY 10010
Telephone: 212-532-0363

A nonprofit organization that provides difficult-to-find AIDS treatments
for people with AIDS.

Compounding Pharmacies

College Pharmacy
Telephone: 800-888-9358

Specializes in the custom compounding of various drug/nutrient preparations. Your physician can contact the pharmacy by calling its toll-free number.

For Your Health Pharmacy
13215 SE 240th Street, Suite A
Kent, WA 98042
Telephone: 800-456-4325

Provides many of the products discussed in this book. Smart drugs purchased will require a prescription from your physician.

The Mail-Order Pharmacy
3170 North Federal Highway, Suite 104B
Lighthouse Point, FL 33064
Telephone: 800-822-5388
Fax: 800-487-1821

Discounts prescriptions to members of the Life Extension Foundation. Your physician should contact Dr. Alan Zimmer for further information on ordering prescriptions.

The Eat Smart, Think Smart Smart-Nutrient Computer Program for Windows

The Eat Smart, Think Smart computer program for Microsoft Windows shows you how to find "smart" amino acids and other smart nutrients in foods, recipes, spices, condiments, and canned and frozen foods. As the first smart-nutrient program for Windows, it can help you find all the vital nutrients in your diet that your brain needs to build its own smart chemicals, such as the neurotransmitters norepinephrine, serotonin, dopamine, and nitric oxide.

Eat Smart, Think Smart will graph the amino-acid content (as well as amino-acid ratios by fixed or variable scale) of foods and recipes, revealing which ones are low in specific essential amino acids. The program also produces a number of easy-to-read graphs and pie charts that let you track your intake of smart nutrients (or cholesterol, saturated fat, protein, calories, and so forth) over time.

The program easily converts units of measure (such as grams, ounces, pounds, teaspoons, and tablespoons) and lets you make "what-if" changes to food quantities and see the nutritional effects of such changes on recipes and menus. It also keeps track of daily notes and recipes and lets you change the number of people your recipes serve as well as the serving sizes. The caloric breakdown of foods and recipes is shown by the percentages of calories, protein, fat, and carbohydrates. There is no limit on the number of foods, recipes, and daily food-intake records the program will manage.

All the graphs and smart-nutrient calculations, including the recipe analyses in this book, were done on the program.

For information on ordering the program, write or phone

Small Planet Systems Corporation
PO Box 4011
Tallahassee, FL 32315
800-852-6007 or 904-224-9004

Publications That Feature Information on Smart Nutrients and Smart Drugs

The publications listed here feature articles on smart nutrients and smart drugs. The newsletters focus on the field of smart nutrition and smart drugs, including information on how to order them. These publications are listed for information purposes only.

If you know of additional publications or newsletters, please write to me at the following address, so I can include them in future editions of this book:

PO Box 69-3912
Norland Branch
Miami, FL 33169

Haas Health Newsletter
PO Box 69-3912
Norland Branch
Miami, FL 33169
Subscription: $24 (United States), $30 (elsewhere)

The *Haas Health Newsletter* is a biannual report on the latest developments in nutrition you can use, including smart nutrients, life-extension products, and an easy-to-understand synopses of important discoveries that can improve the quality of your life.

Longevity
PO Box 3226
Harlan, IA 51593
Telephone: 800-333-2782
Subscription: $17.97 (United States)

Longevity is a monthly magazine that features articles on life extension and staying young, smart nutrients and nootropic drugs, general nutrition, beauty regimens, and high-tech gadgets that can help you do everything from meditating to building a better body.

Mondo 2000
PO Box 10171
Berkeley, CA 94709
Telephone: 510-845-9018
Fax: 510-649-9630
Subscription: $24 (United States), $27 (Canada) $50 (elsewhere)

Mondo 2000 is a monthly magazine targeted at Generation X. Cyberpunks, computer hackers, high techies, virtual-reality freaks, UFO aficionados, research scientists, pop psychologists, and college students will find this unique, avant-garde publication fascinating reading.

Omni
PO Box 3026
Harlan, IA 51593
Telephone: 800-289-6664
Subscription: $17.97 (United States)

Omni covers a wide range of scientific, technological, and political issues for the educated lay reader. Feature articles cover smart drugs and nutrients, life-extension therapies, and interviews with prominent antiaging experts.

Psychology Today
PO Box 51844
Boulder, CO 80321
Subscription: $15.97 (United States)

This monthly magazine features articles on smart nutrients, how foods affect the mind, and how psychotropic drugs affect your life and general pop-psychology features that cover general health, job stress, sexual interests, and family issues.

Citizens for Health Quarterly Newsletter
PO Box 368
Tacoma, WA 98401
Telephone: 800-357-2211 or 206-922-2457
Subscription: $25 (includes membership), $75 (includes subscription
    to *National Fax Network News* for important updates)

This nonprofit consumer watchdog organization provides up-to-date coverage of the FDA's attempts to remove nutritional supplements from the consumer market, apprises readers of pending health legislation, and exposes the real politics behind many of the health decisions made by national health-care organizations. This is a must-have publication for all people concerned with current health-related events. A subscription to the newsletter is automatic with membership in the organization.

Life Extension Report
PO Box 229120
Hollywood, FL 33022
Telephone: 305-966-4886
Subscription: $27 (United States), $33 (elsewhere)

This newsletter is published by the Life Extension Foundation, a distributor of life-extension products, therapies, books, and tapes. Articles deal with smart drugs and nutrients, the FDA's regulatory actions and abuses, and recent developments in the area of antiaging and general health.

Nootropic News Newsletter
PO Box 177
Camarillo, CA 93011
Telephone: 805-379-2666
Subscription: $12 (United States)

This quarterly newsletter is devoted to developments in the field of nootropic drugs and other intelligence-boosting substances. Issues include a brief review of the medical literature, synopses of selected smart drugs, and FDA and congressional actions concerning nootropics.

How to Use Your Computer to Learn More About Research on Smart Nutrients

Two of the most important forces currently shaping the way people can learn about smart-nutrition research and/or talk directly to researchers or people with the same interests is through information networks and database services. Both provide up-to-the-minute information and communication services at a relatively low cost.

If you have a personal computer at home or at the office and a modem, you can learn about the latest (and past) nutritional research, classified by author, title, journal name, or key words, and limit the search to any author, year, topic, language, source, or key word. Most services also list foreign journals and provide abstracts of articles in English. Some information services provide an opportunity to communicate directly with other subscribers (via computer) in a number of countries. Much of the research for this book was initiated using several of the on-line services listed here (check with the services; prices usually vary with time):

America Online, Inc.
8619 Westwood Center Drive
Vienna, VA 22182
Telephone: 800-827-6364
Fax: 703-883-1509

Monthly fee: $7.95 with two free hours, additional time: 10 cents per minute, hourly fee: $5–$10

ClariNet Communications Corp.
5000 Arlington Centre Boulevard
PO Box 20212
Columbus, OH 43220
Telephone: 800-848-8199

ClariNet monthly fee: $35 for a single user; noncommercial home license: $15 per month, 15 users: $52.50; newsbytes only, monthly fee: $10 for a single user, $83 for 100 users; site licenses available.

CompuServe, Inc.
5000 Arlington Centre Boulevard
PO Box 20212
Columbus, OH 43220
Telephone: 800-848-8199
Fax: 614-457-0348

The CompuServe Information Service starter kit: $49.95 ($39.95 if purchased from CompuServe). Monthly fee: $7.95 for unlimited access to 30 basic services with 60 E-mail messages per month at no extra charge, $.15 cents thereafter; access to bulletin boards: 21 cents per minute or $12.60 per hour at 1200 or 2400 baud (bits per second).

DataTimes
14000 Quail Springs Parkway, Suite 450
Oklahoma City, OK 73134
Telephone: 800-642-2525
Fax: 405-751-6400

DataTimes sign-up fee: $85. Monthly charges: $15, with on-line charges of $1.16–$1.91 per minute, or $75, with on-line charges of 69 cents to $1.19 per minute; flat-fee pricing is available.

Delphi
Telephone: 800-544-4005

Delphi's 10/4 plan costs $10 per month for 4 hours on-line; its 20/20 plan costs $20 per month for 20 hours on-line.

Dialog Information Services
3460 Hillview Avenue
Palo Alto, CA 94304
Telephone: 800-334-2564
Fax: 415-858-7069

Dialog sign-up fee: $45; annual fee: $35. Hourly rates: $24–$312 plus per-word charges. Knowledge Index sign-up fee: $40 plus 40 cents per minute (accessible only after hours).

Echo
Telephone: 212-255-3839

Fee: $18 per month ($12.95 for students and the elderly) for 30 hours on-line; additional time: $1 per hour.

Dow Jones & Co.
PO Box 300
Princeton, NJ 08543
Telephone: 800-522-3567
Fax: 609-520-4660

Dow Jones News Retrieval sign-up fee: $29.95. Annual fee: $18 per year after the first year; 60 cents to $2.16 per minute plus download fees.

General Electric Co.
PO Box 6403
Rockville, MD 20859
Telephone: 800-638-9636

GEnie monthly fee: $4.95 plus $18 per hour prime time (8 A.M.–6 P.M., Eastern Standard Time). Bulletin boards: $6 per hour after hours (6 P.M.–8 A.M.)

Mead Data Central, Inc.
PO Box 933
Dayton, OH 45401
Telephone: 800-277-4908
Fax: 513-865-1666

Nexis monthly fee: $50; Nexis and Lexis monthly fee: $125; on-line charges vary, and volume discounts are available.

NewsNet, Inc.
945 Haverford Road
Bryn Mawr, PA 19010
Telephone: 800-952-0122
Fax: 215-527-0388

NewsNet annual fee: $120; hourly fee: $60–$90

Prodigy Services Co.
445 Hamilton Avenue
White Plains, NY 10601
Telephone: 800-776-3449
Fax: 914-684-0278

Prodigy monthly fee: $14.95 for unlimited on-line time.

The Well
Telephone: 415-332-4335

The Well's fees: $15 per month plus $2 per-hour on-line for users within the 415 area code (San Francisco); users outside the 415 area code can access the Well through InterNet or CompuServe; both charge $4 per hour.

Ziff Desktop Information
25 First Street
Cambridge, MA 02141
Telephone: 617-252-5200
Fax: 617-252-5551

ZiffNet and ZiffNet/Mac monthly fee: $2.50 for access to basic services; hourly fee: $12.80–$22.80 for other services.

FDA Survival Guide

If the FDA succeeds in reclassifying the four targeted nutrients/herbs listed below as drugs, effectively removing them from the consumer market and turning them over to the pharmaceutical industry (as prescription "medications"), you'll need to know how to get them—legally—so you can eat smart to think smart.

If the FDA removes this nutrient from the market	*Use this nutritional strategy to obtain the nutrient*
L-arginine	Eat L-arginine-rich snacks between meals, such as 3½ ounces of turkey or chicken breast; ½ cup of dry-roasted soybean nuts; one cup of split peas, lentils, or chick-peas; one cup of low-fat cottage cheese. Take one 2 mg vitamin B_6 capsule.
L-tryptophan (already removed from the market by the FDA)	Eat one ounce of dried sunflower seeds or one banana or drink Lights Out Hot Toddy (recipe in Chapter 6) one hour before retiring.
Coenzyme Q_{10}	Eat a tuna fish sandwich made with white albacore tuna (packed in spring water) mixed with low-fat mayonnaise, on whole-grain bread.
Ma Huang (ephedra)	Use an over-the-counter cold remedy that contains ephedrine (use only as directed, and obtain your physician's approval before using).

Bibliography

Acworth, I. N., During, M. J., Wurtman, R. J. Tyrosine: effects on catecholamine release. *Brain Res Bull,* 1988; 21(3), 474–77.

Agmo, A., and Fernandez, H. Dopamine and sexual behavior in the male rat: A reevaluation. *J. Neural Transm* 1989; 77(1): 21.

Alkadhi, K. A. Endplate channel actions of a hemicholinium-3 analog, DMAE. *Naunyn Schmiedebergs Arch Pharmacol* 1986; 332(3): 230.

Amenta, D., Ferrante, F., Franch, F., and Amenta, F. Effects of long-term Hydergine administration on lipofuscin accumulation in senescent rat brain. *Gerontology* 1988; 34(5–6): 250.

Amenta, F., Cavallotti, C., Franch, F., and Ricci, A. Muscarinic cholinergic receptors in the hippocampus of the aged rat: Effects of long-term Hydergine administration. *Arch Int Pharmacodyn Ther* 1989; 297: 225.

Anderson, I., and Cowen, P. Neuroendocrine responses to L-tryptophan as an index of brain serotonin function: Effect of weight loss. *Adv Exp Med Biol* 1991; 294: 245.

Andrews, L. D., and Brizzee, K. R. Lipofuscin in retinal pigment epithelium of rhesus monkey: Lack of diminution with centrophenoxine treatment. *Neurobiol Aging* 1986; 7(2): 107.

Andriamampandry, C., Freysz, L., Kanfer, J. N., Dreyfus, H., and Massarelli, R. Conversion of ethanolamine, monomethylethanolamine and dimethylethanolamine to choline-containing compounds by neurons in culture and by the rat brain. *Biochem J* 1989; 264(2): 555.

Anger, C., Van, A. H., Hoch, D., and Lawin, P. The influence of ketanserin, droperidol and Hydergine on postoperative hypertension during early recovery following major abdominal surgery. *Acta Anaesthesiol Belg* 1987; 38(2): 153.

Anon. No news is good news. *Science* 1992; 258: 1862.

Arduini, A., Rossi, M., Mancinelli, G., et al. Effect of L-carnitine and acetyl-L-carnitine on the human erythrocyte membrane stability and deformability. *Life Sci* 1990; 47(26): 2395.

Arnold, M. E., Petros, T. V., Beckwith, B. E., Coons, G., and Gorman, N. The effects of caffeine, impulsivity, and sex on memory for word list. *Physiol Behav* 1987; 41(1): 25.

Arrigo, A., Casale, R., Giorgi, I., Guarnaschelli, C., and Zelaschi, F. Effects of intravenous high dose co-dergocrine mesylate ("Hydergine") in elderly patients with severe multi-infarct dementia: A double-blind, placebo-controlled trial. *Curr Med Res Opin* 1989; 11(8): 491.

Asheychik, R., Jackson, T., Baker, H., Ferraro, R., Ashton, T., and Kilgore, J. The efficacy of L-tryptophan in the reduction of sleep disturbance and depressive state in alcoholic patients. *J Stud Alcohol* 1989; 50(6): 525.

Astrup, A., et al. Caffeine: A double-blind, placebo-controlled study of its thermogenic, metabolic, and cardiovascular effects on healthy volunteers. *Amer J of Clin Nut* 1990; 52: 759.

Astrup, A., et al. The effect and safety of an ephedrine/caffeine compound compared with ephedrine, caffeine, and placebo in obese subjects on an energy restricted diet. *Obesity* 1992; 16: 269.

Astrup, A., et al. The effect of ephedrine/caffeine mixture on energy expenditures and body composition in obese women. *Metabolism* 1992; 41: 886.

Astrup, A., and Toubro, S. Thermogenic, metabolic, and cardiovascular responses to ephedrine and caffeine in man. *International Journal of Obesity* 1993; 17 (Suppl 1): S41–S43:

Bacciottini, L., Pellegrine, G. D. E., Bongianni, F., et al. Biochemical and behavioural studies on indole-pyruvic acid: A keto-analogue of tryptophan. *Pharmacol Res Commun* 1987; 19(11): 803.

Baer, L., Jenike, M. A. Hydergine in Alzheimer's disease [letter]. *J Geriatr Psychiatry Neurol* 1991; 4(2): 122.

Baer, R. A. Effects of caffeine on classroom behavior, sustained attention, and a memory task in preschool children. *J Appl Behav Anal* 1987; 20(3): 225.

Bakalian, M. J., and Fernstrom, J. D. Effects of L-tryptophan and other amino acids on electroencephalographic sleep in the rat. *Brain Res* 1990; 528(2): 300.

Baltzell, J. K., Bazer, F. W., Miguel, S. G., and Borum, P. R. The neonatal piglet as a model for human neonatal carnitine metabolism. *J Nutr* 1987; 117(4): 754.

Barja-de-Quiroga, G., Perez-Campo, R., and Lopez-Torres, M. Changes in cerebral antioxidant enzymes, peroxidation, and the glutathione system of frogs after aging and catalase inhibition. *J Neurosci Res* 1990; 26(3): 370.

Bartellini, M., Canale, D., Izzo, P. L., Giorgi, P. M., Meschini, P., and Meschini, F. G. F. L-carnitine and acetylcarnitine in human sperm with normal and reduced motility. *Acta Eur Fertil* 1987; 18(1): 29.

Battino, M., Fato, R., Parenti, C. G., and Lenaz, G. Coenzyme Q can control the efficiency of oxidative phosphorylation. *Int J Tissue React* 1990; 12(3): 137.

Bazzato, G., Coli, U., Landini, S., et al. Myasthenia-like syndrome after D, L- but not L-carnitine. *Lancet* 1981; 1(8231).

Benzi, G., Marzatico, F., Pastoris, O., and Villa, R. F. Relationship between aging, drug treatment and the cerebral enzymatic antioxidant system. *Exp Gerontol* 1989; 24(2): 137.

Benzi, G., Pastoris, O., Marzatico, F., and Villa, R. F. Cerebral enzyme antioxidant system. Influence of aging and phosphatidylcholine. *J Cereb Blood Flow Metab* 1989; 9(3): 373.

Benzi, G., Pastoris, O., Marzatico, F., Villa, R. F., Dagani, F., and Curti, D. The mitochondrial electron transfer alteration as a factor involved in the brain aging. *Neurobiol Aging* 1992; 13(3): 361.

Bertelli, A., and Ronca, G. Carnitine and coenzyme Q_{10}: Biochemical properties and functions, synergism and complementary action. *Int J Tissue React* 1990; 12(3): 183.

Bertoni, F. C., Giuli, C., Pieri, C., et al. The effect of chronic Hydergine treatment on the plasticity of synaptic junctions in the dentate gyrus of aged rats. *J Gerontol* 1987; 42(5): 482.

Bes, A., Dupui, P., Guell, A., Bessoles, G., and Geraud, G. Pharmacological exploration of dopamine hypersensitivity in migraine patients. *Int J Clin Pharmacol Res* 1986; 6(3): 189.

Beyer, R. E. The participation of coenzyme Q in free radical production and antioxidation. *Free Radic Biol Med* 1990; 8(6): 545.

Bindoli, A., Rigobello, M. P., and Deble, D. J. Biochemical and toxicological properties of the oxidation products of catecholamines. *Free Radic Biol Med* 1992; 13: 391.

Bohles, H., Richter, K., Wagner, T. E., and Schafer, H. Decreased serum carnitine in valproate induced Reye syndrome. *Eur J Pediatr* 1982; 139(3): 185.

Boissonneault, G. A., Hennig, B., Wang, Y., and Wood, C. L. Aging and endothelial barrier function in culture: Effects of chronic exposure to fatty acid hydroperoxides and vitamin E. *Mech Ageing Dev* 1990; 56(1): 1.

Boldyrev, A. A., Dupin, A. M., Bunin, A., Babizhaev, M. A., and Severin S. E. The antioxidative properties of carnosine, a natural histidine containing dipeptide. *Biochem Int* 1987; 15(6): 1105.

Boldyrev, A. A., and Severin, S. E. The histidine-containing dipeptides, carnosine and anserine: Distribution, properties and biological significance. *Adv Enzyme Regul* 1990; 30: 175.

Bonavita, E. Neuropsychological study of the senile brain during and after single and combined treatment with deanol and citicoline. *Clin Ther* 1986; 117(5): 387.

Boulat, O., Waldmeier, P., and Maitre, L. 3,4-Dihydroxyphenylacetic acid (DOPAC) as an index of noradrenaline turnover: Effects of Hydergine and vincamine. *J Neural Transm Gen Sect* 1990; 82(3): 181.

Bowyer, B. A., Miles, J. M., Haymond, M. W., and Fleming, C. R. L-carnitine therapy in home parenteral nutrition patients with abnormal liver tests and low plasma carnitine concentrations. *Gastroenterology* 1988; 94(2): 434.

Brackett, N. L., Iuvone, P. M., and Edwards, D. A. Midbrain lesions, dopamine and male sexual behavior. *Behav Brain Res* 1986; 20(2): 231.

Branconnier, R. The efficiency of the cerebral metabolic enhancers in the treatment of senile dementia. *Psychopharmacol Bull* 1983; 19(2): 212.

Bucci, L., Hickson, J. F., Wolinsky, I., et al. Ornithine supplementation and insulin release in bodybuilders. *Int J Sports Nutr* 1992; 2: 287.

Cai, N. [Treatment of 37 cases of tardive dyskinesia by deanol]. *Chung Hua Shen Ching Ching Shen Ko Tsa Chih* 1985; 18(4): 234.

Callaway, E., Halliday, R., and Naylor, H. Cholinergic activity and constraints on information processing. *Biol Psychol* 1992; 33(1): 1.

Cand, F., and Verdetti, J. Superoxide dismutase, glutathione peroxidase, catalase, and lipid peroxidation in the major organs of the aging rats. *Free Radic Biol Med* 1989; 7(1): 59.

Cayley, A. C. D., Macpherson, A., and Wedgewood, J. Sinus bradycardia following treatment with Hydergine for cerebrovascular insufficiency. *Br Med J* 1975; 4(5993): 384.

Cederblad, G., and Gothenburg, S. Effect of diet on plasma carnitine levels and urinary carnitine excretion in humans. *Am J Clin Nutr* 1987; 45(4): 725.

Chen, T. S., Richie, J. P., Jr., and Lang, C. A. The effect of aging on glutathione and cysteine levels in different regions of the mouse brain. *Proc Soc Exp Biol Med* 1989; 190(4): 399.

Chiarenza, G. A., Ragaini, C., and Guareschi, C. A. The acute and chronic administrations of piracetam affect the movement-related brain macropotentials. *Int J Psychophysiol* 1990; 8(3): 223.

Chrisp, P., Mammen, G. J., and Sorkin, E. M. Selegiline: A review of its pharmacology, symptomatic benefits, and protective potential in Parkinson's disease. *Drugs Aging* 1991; 1: 228.

Clair, F., Caillat, S., Soufir, J. C., et al. Myasthenia-like syndrome induced by DL-carnitine in a chronic haemodialysis patient. *Presse Med* 1984; 13(18): 1154.

Clark, B. J., Bucher, T., and Waite, R. Analysis of the cardiovascular effects of co-derocrine (Hydergine). *J Pharmacol* 1985; 3: 101.

Clark, J. T., Gabriel, S. M., Simpkins, J. W., Kalra, S. P., and Kalra, P. S. Chronic morphine and testosterone treatment. Effects on sexual behavior and dopamine metabolism in male rats. *Neuroendocrinol* 1988; 48(1): 97.

Cohen, M. R., Pary, R., and Burns, R. Hydergine for schizophrenia [letter]. *J Clin Psychiatry* 1987; 48(1): 39.

Contijoch, A. M., Johnson, A. L., and Advis, J. P. Norepinephrine-stimulated in vitro release of luteinizing hormone-releasing hormone (LHRH) from median eminence tissue is facilitated by inhibition of LHRH-degrading activity in hens. *Biol Reprod* 1990; 42(2): 222.

Corbucci, G. G., Gasparetto, A., Antonelli, M., et al. Effects of L-carnitine administration on mitochondrial electron transport activity present in human muscle during circulatory shock. *Int J Clin Pharmacol Res* 1985; 5(4): 237.

Corbucci, G. G., Gasparetto, A., Antonelli, M., Bufi, M., and De, B. R. A. Changes in the levels of coenzyme Q homologues, alpha-tocopherol and malondialdehyde in human tissue during the course of circulatory shock. *J Pediatr* 1987; 110(2): 216.

Corbucci, G. G., Montanari, G., Mancinelli, G., and Diddio, S. Metabolic effects induced by L-carnitine and propionyl-L-carnitine in human hypoxic muscle tissue during exercise. *Int J Clin Pharmacol Res* 1990; 10(3): 197.

Crawley, J. N., and Wenk, G. L. Co-existence of galanin and acetylcholine: Is galanin involved in memory processes and dementia? *Trends Neurosci* 1989; 12(8): 278.

Cress, A. P., Fraker, P. J., and Bieber, L. L. Carnitine and acylcarnitine levels of human peripheral blood lymphocytes and mononuclear phagocytes. *Biochim Biophys Acta* 1989; 992(2): 135.

Crofford, L. J., Rader, J. I., Dalakas, M. C., et al. L-tryptophan implicated in human eosinophilia-myalgia syndrome causes fascilitis and perimyositis in the Lewis rat. *J Clin Invest* 1990; 86(5): 1757.

Czyzewski, K. [Various aspects of lipid metabolism in the human body with special reference to the role of carnitine]. *Wiad Lek* 1989; 42(13–15): 884.

D'Andrea, G., Cananzi, A. R., Grigoletto, F., et al. The effect of dopamine receptor agonists on prolactin secretion in childhood migraine. *Headache* 1988; 28(5): 354.

Daly, P. A., Krieger, D. R., Dulloo, A. G., et al. Ephedrine, caffeine, and aspirin; safety and efficacy for treatment of human obesity. *International Journal of Obesity* 1993, 17 (Suppl 1): S73–78.

Datta, K. D., Evenson, R. C., Gannon, P. J., and Dick, E. P. Efficacy of oral Hydergine (ergoloid mesylates) in alcohol related encephalopathy. *Prog Neuropsychopharmacol Biol Psychiatry* 1987; 11(1): 87.

De, G. D., Mezzina, C., Fiaschi, A., et al. Myasthenia due to carnitine treatment. *J Neurol Sci* 1980; 46(3): 365.

de la Morena, E. Efficacy of CDP-choline in the treatment of senile alterations in memory. *Ann N.Y. Acad Sci* 1991; 640: 233.

de-Haan, J. B., Newman, J. D., Kola, I. Cu/Zn superoxide dismutase mRNA and enzyme activity, and susceptibility to lipid peroxidation, increases with aging in murine brains. *Brain Res Mol Brain Res* 1992; 13(3): 179.

Deana, R., Indino, M., Rigoni, F., and Foresta, C. Effect of L-carnitine on motility and acrosome reaction of human spermatozoa. *Arch Androl* 1988; 21(3): 147.

Del-Maestro, R., and McDonald, W. Distribution of superoxide dismutase, glutathione peroxidase and catalase in developing rat brain. *Mech Ageing Dev* 1987; 41(1–2): 29.

Delahunty, D. A. A possible role of oxygen metabolism in the evolution of the human life span: Antioxidants and aging (genetics, Alzheimer's disease, aging, oxygen radicals). *Dai* 1984; 45(07).

Di, D. S., Frerman, F. E., Rimoldi, M., Rinaldo, P., Taroni, F., and Wisemann, U. N. Systemic carnitine deficiency due to lack of electron transfer flavoprotein: Ubiquinone oxidoreductase. *Neurol* 1986; 36(7): 957.

Di, I. M., Wilsher, C. R., Blank, M. S., et al. The effects of piracetam in children with dyslexia. *J Clin Psychopharmacol* 1985 5(5): 272.

Dominiak, R., and Weidinger, G. [Therapy comparison between the combination Hydergine/nifedipine and nifedipine alone in patients with isolated systolic hypertension]. *Med Klin* 1991; 86(1): 15.

Dowson, J. H. Quantitative studies of the effects of aging, meclofenoxate, and dihydroergotoxine on intraneuronal lipopigment accumulation in the rat. *Exp Gerontol* 1985; 20(6): 333.

Dowson, J. H. Neuronal lipopigment: A marker for cognitive impairment and long-term effects of psychotropic drugs. *Br J Psychiatry* 1989; 155: 1.

Dravid, A. R., and Hiestand, P. Deficits in cholinergic enzyme activities in septo-temporal regions of the senescent rat hippocampus, and in the forebrain of aged mice: Effect of chronic Hydergine treatment. *J Pharmacol* 1985; 3: 25.

Dulloo, A. The do-do pill: Potentiation of the thermogenic effects of ephedrine by methylxanthines. *Pro Nutr Soc* 1985; 44: 16.

Dulloo, A. Potentiation of the thermogenic antiobesity effects of ephedrine by dietary methylxanthines: Adenosine antagonism or phosphodiesterase inhibition? *Metabolism* 1992; 41: 1233.

Dulloo, A., et al. Aspirin as a promoter of ephedrine-induced thermogenesis: Potential use in the treatment of obesity. *Amer J Clin Nut* 1987; 45: 564.

Dulloo, A., and Miller, D. S. The thermogenic properties of ephedrine/methylxanthine mixtures: Human studies. *Int J Obesity* 1986; 10: 467.

Dulloo, A., and Miller, D. S. Ephedrine, caffeine, and aspirin: Over-the-counter drugs that interact to stimulate thermogenesis in the obese. *Nutrition* 1989; 5: 7.

Durkin, T. Central cholinergic pathways and learning and memory processes: Presynaptic aspects. *Comp Biochem Physiol* [a] 1989; 93(1): 273.

Edwards, D. J., Sorisio, D. A., and Knopf, S. Effects of the beta 2-adrenoceptor agonist clenbuterol on tyrosine and tryptophan in plasma and brain of the rat. *Biochem Pharmacol* 1989; 38(18): 2957.

El, S. A., El, S. M., Darwish, A. K., Davies, T., Griffin, K., and Keshavan, M. S. Hydergine effect on prolactin and reaction time in dementia [letter]. *Biol Psychiatry* 1986; 21(12): 1229.

Elmadfa, I., Both, B. N., Sierakowski, B., and Steinhagen, T. E. [Significance of vitamin E in aging]. *J Gerontol* 1986; 19(3): 206.

Erikson, G. C., Hager, L. B., Houseworth, C., Dungan, J., Petros, T., and Beckwith, B. E. The effects of caffeine on memory for word lists. *Physiol Behav* 1985; 35(1): 47.

Ermini, M. The effects of Hydergine on neurotransmitters. *Br J Clin Pract Symp Suppl* 1985; 39: 11.

Estrada, C., Bready, J., Berliner, J., and Cancilla, P. A. Choline uptake by cerebral capillary endothelial cells in culture. *J. Neurochem* 1990; 54(5): 1467.

Farooqui, M. Y., Day, W. W., and Zamorano, D. M. Glutathione and lipid peroxidation in the aging rat. *Comp Biochem Physiol* [b] 1987; 88(1): 177.

Feller, A. G., and Rudman, D. Role of carnitine in human nutrition. *J Nutr* 1988; 118(5): 541.

Fernandez, R. J., De, M. R., Hernandez, M. L., Cebeira, M., and Ramos, J. A. Comparisons between brain dopaminergic neurons of juvenile and aged rats: Sex-related differences. *Mech Ageing Dev* 1992; 63(1): 45.

Finnegan, K. T., Ricaurte, G. A., Ritchie, L. D., Irwin, I., Peroutka, S. J., and Langston, J. W. Orally administered MDMA causes a long-term depletion of serotonin in rat brain. *Brain Res* 1988; 447(1): 141.

Fischer, J. C., Ruitenbeek, W., Gabreels, F. J., et al. A mitochondrial encephalomyopathy: The first case with an established defect at the level of coenzyme Q. *Neurol* 1986; 36(7): 957.

Fischer, W., Kittner, H., and Schubert, S. [The action of piracetam, meclofenoxate and vinpocetine in comparative disease models in mice]. *Pharmazie* 1991; 46(5): 359.

Flood, J. F., Smith, G. E., and Cherkin, A. Hydergine enhances memory in mice. *J Pharmacol* 1985; 3: 39.

Folkers, K., Langsjoen, P., Willis, R., et al. Lovastatin decreases coenzyme Q levels in humans. *Proc Natl Acad Sci U.S.A* 1990; 87(22): 8931.

Fregly, J. J., Sumners, C., and Cade, J. R. Effect of chronic dietary treatment with L-tryptophan on the maintenance of hypertension in spontaneously hypertensive rats. *Can J Physiol Pharmacol* 1989; 67(6): 656.

Fujiwara, F., Todo, S., and Imashuku, S. Antitumor effect of gamma-linolenic acid on cultured human neuroblastoma cells. *Int J Tissue React* 1986; 8(5): 421.

Ganguly, R., and Waldman, R. H. Macrophage functions in aging effects of vitamin C deficiency. *Allerg Immunol* (Leipzig) 1985; 31(1): 37.

Gattaz, W. F., Behrens, S., De, V. J., and Hafner, H. [Estradiol inhibits dopamine mediated behavior in rats—an animal model of sex-specific differences in schizophrenia]. *Fortschr Neurol Psychiatr* 1992; 60(1): 8.

George, C. F., Millar, T. W., Hanly, P. J., and Kryger, M. H. The effect of L-tryptophan on daytime sleep latency in normals: Correlation with blood levels. *Sleep* 1989; 12(4): 345.

Gerlo, E. A., Schoors, D. F., and Dupont, A.G. Age- and sex-related differences for the urinary excretion of norepinephrine, epinephrine, and dopamine in adults. *Clin Chem* 1991; 37(6): 875.

Givens, B. S., Olton, D.S., and Crawley, J. N. Galanin in the medial septal area impairs working memory. *Brain Res* 1992; 582(1): 71.

Gjessing, L. R., Lunde, H. A., Mrkrid, L., Lenney, J. F., and Sjaastad, O. Inborn errors of carnosine and homocarnosine metabolism. *J Neural Transm Suppl* 1990; 29: 91.

Golan, R., Shalev, D. P., Wasserzug, O., Weissenberg, R., and Lewin, L. M. Influence of various substrates on the acetylcarnitine: carnitine ratio in motile and immotile human spermatozoa. *J Reprod Fertil* 1986; 78(1): 287.

Goshima, Y., Nakamura, S., and Misu, Y. L-dihydroxyphenylalanine methyl ester is a potent competitive antagonist of the L-dihydroxyphenylalanine-induced facilitation of the evoked release of endogenous norepinephrine from rat hypothalamic slices. *J Pharmacol Exp Ther* 1991; 258(2): 466.

Gramatte, T., Wustmann, C., Schmidt, J., and Fischer, H. D. Effects of nootropic drugs on some behavioural and biochemical changes after early postnatal hypoxia in the rat. *Biomed Biochim Acta* 1986; 45(8): 1075.

Greenberg, S., and Frishman, W. H. Co-enzyme Q_{10}: A new drug for cardiovascular disease. *J Clin Pharmacol* 1990; 30(7): 596.

Group, T. P. S., Effects of tocopherol and deprenyl on the progression of disability in early Parkinson's disease. *New Engl J Med* 1993; 328(3): 176.

Guze, B. H., and Baxter, L. R. J., The serotonin syndrome: Case responsive to propranolol. *J Clin Psychopharmacol* 1986; 6(2): 119.

Haeckel, R., Colic, D., Binder, L., and Oellerich, M. Stimulation of glucose metabolism in human blood cells by inhibitors of carnitine-dependent fatty acid transport. *J Clin Chem Clin Biochem* 1990; 28(5): 329.

Hafner, H., Behrens, S., De, V. J., and Gattaz, W. F. An animal model for the effects of estradiol on dopamine-mediated behavior: implications for sex differences in schizophrenia. *Psychiatry Res* 1991; 38(2): 125.

Haider, S. S., and Kashyap, S. K. Vanadium intoxication inhibits sulfhydryl groups and glutathione in the rat brain. *Ind Health* 1989; 27(1): 23.

Hajak, G., Huether, G., Blanke, J., et al. The influence of intravenous L-tryptophan on plasma melatonin and sleep in men. *Pharmacopsychiatry* 1991; 24(1): 17.

Halliwell, B., and Gutteridge, J. M. C. Oxygen radicals and the nervous system. *Trens Neurosci* 1985; 8: 22.

Hamagishi, Y., Murata, S., Kamei, H., Oki, T., Adachi, O., and Ameyama, M. New biological properties of pyrroloquinoline quinone and its related compounds: inhibition of chemiluminescence, lipid peroxidation and rat paw edema. *J Pharmacol Exp Ther,* 1990; 255(3), 980-5.

Hamilton, J. W., Li, B. U., Shug, A. L., and Olsen, W. A. Carnitine transport in human intestinal biopsy specimens. Demonstration of an active transport system. *Gastroenterol* 1986; 91(1): 10.

Hamilton, J. J., and Hahn, P. Carnitine and carnitine esters in rat bile and human duodenal fluid. *Can J Physiol Pharmacol* 1987; 65(9): 1816.

Hansen, S., Harthon, C., Wallin, E., Lofberg, L., and Svensson, K. Mesotelencephalic dopamine system and reproductive behavior in the female rat: Effects of ventral tegmental 6-hydroxydopamine lesions on maternal and sexual responsiveness. *Behav Neurosci* 1991; 105(4): 588.

Hasselmo, M. E., Anderson, B. P., and Bower, J. M. Cholinergic modulation of cortical associative memory function. *J Neurophysiol* 1992; 67(5): 1230.

Haug, B. A., and Holzgraefe, M. Orofacial and respiratory tardive dyskinesia: Potential side effects of 2-dimethylaminoethanol (deanol)? *Eur Neurol* 1991; 31(6): 423.

Hazelton, G. A Glutathione metabolism during the life span with emphasis on senescence. *Dai* 1982; 43(07).

Herdon, J. J., and Wilson, C. A. Changes in hypothalamic dopamine D-2 receptors during sexual maturation in male and female rats. *Brain Res* 1985; 343(1): 151.

Heyes, M. P., and Markey, S. P. Quantification of quinolinic acid in rat brain, whole blood, and plasma by gas chromatography and negative chemical ionization mass spectrometry: Effects of systemic L-tryptophan administration on brain and blood quinolinic acid concentrations. *Anal Biochem* 1988; 174(1): 349.

Hindmarch, I., et al. The effects of an ergot alkaloid derivative (Hydergine) on aspects of psychomotor performance, arousal, and cognitive processing ability. *J Clin Pharmacol* 1979 (Nov.–Dec.): 726.

Hollander, D., and Dadufalza, V. Lymphatic and portal absorption of vitamin E in aging rats. *Dig Dis Sci* 1989; 34(5): 768.

Holme, E., Jacobson, C. E., Nordin, I, et al. Carnitine deficiency induced by pivampicillin and pivmecillinam therapy. *Lancel* 1989; 2(8661): 469.

Holmes, E. W., and Kahn, S. E. Tryptophan distribution and metabolism in experimental chronic renal insufficiency. *Exp Mol Pathol* 1987; 46(1): 89.

Holt, I. J., Harding, A. E., Cooper, J. M., et al. Impaired mitochondrial beta-oxidation in a patient with an abnormality of the respiratory chain: Studies in skeletal muscle mitochondria. *J Clin Invest* 1990; 85(5): 177.

Huber, F., Koberle, S., Prestele, H., and Spiegel, R. Effects of long-term ergoloid mesylates ("Hydergine") administration in healthy pensioners: 5-year results. *Curr Med Res Opin* 1986; 10(4): 256.

Hull, E. M., Bazzett, T. J., Warner, R. K., Eaton, R. C., and Thompson, J. T. Dopamine receptors in the entral tegmental area modulate male sexual behavior in rats. *Brain Res* 1990; 512(1): 1.

Idrobo, F. Mostofsky, D. I., and Nandy, K. Acute effects of centrophenoxine short term administration on counting behavior in rats. *Int J Neurosci* 1988; 42(3–4): 309.

Idzikowski, C., Cowen, P. J., Nutt, D., and Mills, F. J. The effects of chronic ritanserin treatment on sleep and the neuroendocrine response to L-tryptophan. *Psychopharmacol* (Berlin) 1987; 93(4): 416.

Idzikowski, C., and Oswald, I. Interference with human memory by an antibiotic. *Psychopharmacol* 1983; 79(2): 2.

Ihara, Y, Namba, R., Kuroda, S., Sato, T., and Shirabe, T. Mitochondrial encephalomyopathy (MELAS): Pathological study and successful therapy with coenzyme Q_{10} and idebenone. *J Neurol Sci* 1989; 90(3): 263.

Ikeda, Y. [Aging-induced changes of acetylcholine and choline contents in cerebrospinal fluid and memory function]. *Yakubutsu Seishin Kodo* 1990; 10(3): 369.

Imagawa, M. Low erythrocyte coenzyme Q_{10} level in schizophrenic patients. *Jpn J Psychiatry Neurol* 1989; 43(2): 143.

Imagawa, M., Naruse, S., Tsuji, S., Fujioka, A., and Yamaguchi, H. Coenzyme Q_{10}, iron, and vitamin B_6 in genetically-confirmed Alzheimer's disease [letter]. *Lancet* 1992; 340(8820): 671.

Introini, C. I. B., and Baratti, C. M. Memory-modulatory effects of centrally acting noradrenergic drugs: Possible involvement of brain cholinergic mechanisms. *Behav Neural Biol* 1992; 57(3): 248.

Izumiyama, K., and Kogure, K. Effect of dihydroergotoxine mesylate (Hydergine) on delayed neuronal death in the gerbil hippocampus. *Acta Neurol Scand* 1988; 78(3): 214.

Jaedig, S., and Henningsen, N. C. Increased metabolic rate in obese women after ingestion of potassium, magnesium- and phosphate-enriched orange juice or injection of ephedrine. *Int J Obes,* 1991; 15(6), 429–36.

James, I. M. The clinical pharmacology of dihydroergotoxine mesylate (Hydergine). *Br J Clin Pract Symp Suppl* 1985; 39: 21.

Jamnicky, B., Slijepcevic, M., Hadzija, M., Juretic, D., and Borcic, O. Tryptophan content in serum and brain of long-term insulin-treated diabetic rats. *Acta Diabetol Lat* 1991; 28(1): 11.

Jaton, A. L., and Vigouret, J. M. Effects of Hydergine and its components on Lashley maze acquisition rats. *J Pharmacol* 1985; 3: 51.

Jimenez, C. N. J., and Amoros, R. L M. [Hydergine in pathology of the inner ear]. *An Otorrinolaringol Ibero Am* 1990; 17(1): 85.

Johnson, D. A., Ulus, I. H., and Wurtman, R. J. Caffeine potentiates the enhancement by choline of striatal acetylcholine release. *Life Sci,* 1992; 51(20), 1597–601.

Juorio, A. V., Li, X. M., Gonzalez, A., Chedrese, P. J., and Murphy, B. D., Effects of active immunization against gonadotrophin-releasing hormone on the concentrations of noradrenaline, dopamine, 5-hydroxytryptamine and some of their metabolites in the brain and sexual organs of male rats. *Neuroendocrinol* 1991; 54(1): 49.

Kajal, S., and Moudgal, R. P. Dopamine and norepinephrine in the diencephalon of ovariectomized and sham-operated hens around sexual maturity. *Zentralbl Veterinarmed* [a] 1987; 34(2): 113.

Kaneko, S., Takahashi, H., and Satoh, M. The use of Xenopus oocytes to evaluate drugs affecting brain Ca2+ channels: Effects of bifemelane and several nootropic agents. *Eur J Pharmacol* 1990; 189(1): 51.

Kato, T., Yoneda, S., Kako, T., Koketsu, M., Hayano, I., and Fujinami, T. Reduction in blood viscosity by treatment with coenzyme Q_{10} in patients with ischemic heart disease. *Int J Clin Pharmacol Ther Toxicol* 1990; 28(3): 123.

Katrib, K., Adlouni, A. H., and Ferard, G. Carnitine in human polymorphonuclear leukocytes, mononuclear cells, and platelets. *Am J Clin Nutr* 1987; 46(5): 734.

Katts, G. R., et al. The short term therapeutic efficacy of treating obesity with a plan of improved nutrition and moderate caloric restriction. *Curr Ther Res* 1992, 51: 261–274.

Katz, M. L., and Robison, W. G. J. Light and aging effects on vitamin E in the retina and retinal pigment epithelium. *Vision Ress* 1987; 27(11): 1875.

Kay, M. M., Bosman, G. J., Shapiro, S. S., Bendich, A., and Bassel, P. S. Oxidation as a possible mechanism of cellular aging: Vitamin E deficiency causes premature aging and IgG binding to erythrocytes. *Proc Natl Acad Sci U.S.A.* 1986; 83(8): 2463.

Kelly, S. J., and Franklin, K. B. An increase in tryptophan in brain may be a general mechanism for the effect of stress on sensitivity to pain. *Neuropharmacol* 1985; 24(11): 1019.

Kho, T. L, Kengen, R., Leunissen, K. M., Teule, J., and Van, H. J. P. Hydergine and reversibility of cyclosporin nephrotoxicity [letter]. *Lancet* 1986; 2(8503): 394.

Kim, S. J., Lee, K. O., Takamiya, S. and Capaldi, R. A. Mitochondrial myopathy involving ubiquinol-cytochrome c oxidoreductase (complex III) identified by immunoelectron microscopy. *Biochim Biophys Acta* 1987; 894(2): 270.

Kirchgessner, M., Steinhart, H., and Kreuzer, M. [Amino acid pattern in the bodies and several organs of broilers fed different provisions with tryptophan and neutral amino acids]. *Arch Tierernahr* 1988; 38(10): 905.

Kita, K., Oya, H., Gennis R. B., Ackrell, B. A., and Kasahara, M. Mitochondrial complex I deficiency in Parkinson's disease. *J Neurochem* 1990; 54(3): 823.

Knoll, J., Dallo, J., and Yen, T. T. Striatal dopamine, sexual activity and lifespan. Longevity in rats treated with (-)deprenyl. *Life Sci* 1989; 45(6): 525.

Kobayashi, A., Watanabe, H., Fujisawa, S., Yamamoto, T., and Yamazaki, N. Effects of L-carnitine and palmitoylcarnitine on membrane fluidity of human erythrocytes. *Biochim Biophys Acta* 1989; 986(1): 83.

Kobayashi, M., Morishita, H., Sugiyama, N., et al. Two cases of NADH-coenzyme Q reductase deficiency: Relationship to MELAS syndrome. *J Pediatr* 1987; 110(2): 223.

Koeppen, D. Memory and benzodiazepines: Animal and human studies with 1,4-benzodiazepines and clobazam (1,5-benzodiazepine). *Drug Dev Res* 1984; 4(5): 555.

Koga, Y., Nonaka, I., Kobayashi, M., Tojyo, M., and Nihei, K. Findings in muscle in complex I (NADH coenzyme Q reductase) deficiency. *Ann Neurol* 1988; 24(6): 749.

Koga, Y., Nonaka, I., Kobayashi, M., Tojyo, M., and Nihei, K. Muscle coenzyme Q deficiency in familial mitochondrial encephalomyopathy. *Proc Natl Acad Sci U.S.A.* 1989; 86(7): 2379.

Koistinaho, J., Alho, H., and Hervonen A. Effect of vitamin E and selenium supplement on the aging peripheral neurons of the male Sprague-Dawley rat. *Mech Ageing Dev* 1990; 51(1): 63.

Kolbinger, W., Trepel, M., Beyer, C., Pilgrim, C., and Reisert, I. The influence of genetic sex on sexual differentiation of diencephalic dopaminergic neurons in vitro and in vivo. *Brain Res* 1991; 544(2): 349.

Kotagal, S., Peterson, P. L., Martens, M. E., Lee, C. P., Nigro, M., and Archer, C. R. Impaired NADH-CoQ reductase activity in a child with moyamoya syndrome. *Pediatr Neurol* 1988; 4(4): 241.

Kotagal, S., Peterson, P. L., Martens, M. E., Lee, C. P., Nigro, M., and Archer, C. R. Coenzyme Q in serum and muscle of 5 patients with Kearns-Sayre syndrome and 12 patients with ophthalmoplegia plus. *J Neurol* 1989; 236(2): 97.

Kris, M. G., Gralla, R. J., Tyson, L. B., et al. Phase I pharmacologic study of the serotonin antagonist GR-C507/75 (GR38032F) when used as an antiemetic. *Pro Am Soc Clin Oncol* 1988 (1099).

Kukstas, L. A., Domec, C., Bascles, L., et al. Different expression of the two dopaminergic D2 receptors, D2415 and D2444, in two types of lactotroph each characterised by their response to dopamine, and modification of expression by sex steroids. *Endocrinol* 1991; 129(2): 1101.

Lachica, E., Vallanueva, E., and Luna, A. Regional distribution of total lipids, free fatty acids and free carnitine in human heart. *Rev Esp Fisiol* 1988; 44(4): 401.

Langemann, H., Kabiersch, A., and Newcombe, J. Measurement of low-molecular-weight antioxidants, uric acid, tyrosine and tryptophan in plaques and white matter from patients with multiple sclerosis. *Eur Neurol* 1992; 32(5): 248.

Langsjoen, P. H., and Folkers, K. A six-year clinical study of therapy of cardio-myopathy with coenzyme Q_{10}. *Int J Tissue React* 1990; 12(3): 169.

Langsjoen, P. H., and Folkers, K. Long-term efficacy and safety of coenzyme Q_{10} therapy for idiopathic dilated cardiomyopathy. *Am J Cardiol* 1990; 65(7): 521.

Langsjoen, P. H., Folkers, K., Lyson, K., Muratsu, K., and Lyson, T., Pronounced increase of survival of patients with cardiomyopathy when treated with coen-zyme Q_{10} and conventional therapy. *Int J Tissue React* 1990; 12(3): 163.

Lavene, D., Humbert, H., Kiechel, J. R., Ducreuzet, C., Lajoie, D., and Guillevin, L. Hydergine pharmacokinetics in the elderly. *J Pharmacol* 1985; 3: 135.

Le, P. L. M., Rapin, J. R., Duterte, D., Galiez, V., and Lamproglou, I. Learning and cholinergic neurotransmission in old animals: The effect of Hydergine. *J Pharmacol* 1985; 3: 57.

Lennon, D. L., Shrago, E. R., Madden, M., Nagle, F. J., and Hanson, P. Dietary carnitine intake related to skeletal muscle and plasma carnitine concentrations in adult men and women. *Am J Clin Nutr* 1986; 43(2): 234.

Linden, C. H., Vellman, W. P., and Rumack, B. Yohimbine: A new street drug. *Ann Emerg Med* 1985; 14(10): 1002.

Littarru, G. P., Lippa, S., De, S. P., and Oradei, A. In vitro effect of different ubiquinones on the scavenging of biologically generated O2- *Drugs Exp Clin Res* 1985; 11(8): 529.

Littaru, G. P., Lippa, S., De, S. P., and Oradei, A. In vitro effect of different ubiquinones on the scavenging of biologically generated O2- *Prostaglandins Leukot Med* 1986; 23(2–3): 311.

Littarru, G. P., Lippa, S., Oradei, A., and Serino, F. Coenzyme Q_{10}: Blood levels and metabolic demand. *Int J Tissue React* 1990; 12(3): 145.

Lohr, J., and Acara, M. Effect of dimethylaminoethanol, an inhibitor of betaine production, on the disposition of choline in the rat kidney. *J Pharmacol Exp Ther* 1990; 252(1): 154.

Loke, W. H. Effects of caffeine on mood and memory. *Physiol Behav* 1988; 44(3): 367.

Loke, W. H., Hinrichs, J. V., and Ghoneim, M. M. Caffeine and diazepam: Separate and combined effects on mood, memory, and psychomotor perfor-mance. *Psychopharmacol* (Berlin) 1985; 87(3): 344.

Lombard, K. A., Olson, A. L., Nelson, S. E., and Rebouche, C. J. Carnitine status of lactoovovegetarians and strict vegetarian adults and children. *Am J Clin Nutr* 1989; 50(2): 301.

Lopez, J. R., Briceno, L. E., Cordovez, G., Sanchez, V., and Linares, N. Intracellu-lar free [Ca2+] in human skeletal muscle with myopathic carnitine deficiency. *Gen Physiol Biophys* 1989; 8(2): 91.

Lopez-Torres, M., Perez-Campo, R., Fernandez, A., Barba, C., and Barja-de-Quiroga, G. Brain glutathione reductase induction increases early survival and decreases lipofuscin accumulation in aging frogs. *J Neurosci Res* 1993; 34(2): 233.

Louilot, A., Gonzalez, M. J. L., Guadalupe, T., and Mas, M. Sex-related olfactory stimuli induce a selective increase in dopamine release in the nucleus accumbens of male rats: A voltammetric study. *Brain Res* 1991; 553(2): 313.

Lucki, I., Rickels, K., Giesecke, M. A., and Geller, A. Differential effects of the anxiolytic drugs, diazepam and buspirone on memory function. *Br J Clin Pharmacol* 1987; 23(2): 207.

Luderer, U., and Schwartz, N. B. Sex differences in acute luteinizing hormone responses to gonadectomy remain after progesterone antagonist and dopamine agonist treatment. *Biol Reprod* 1991; 45(6): 918.

Lysiak, S. W. [The physiological role of L-carnitine in the human body: Causes and effects of its deficiency]. *Pol Tyg Lek* 1988; 43(10): 337.

Maccari, F., and Hulsmann, W. C. (Acyl)carnitine distribution between plasma, erythrocytes, and leukocytes in human blood [letter]. *Clin Chem* 1989; 35(4): 711.

Maegawa, H., Katsube, N., Okegawa, T., Aishita, H., and Kawasaki, A. Arginine-vasopressin fragment 4-9 stimulates the acetylcholine release in hippocampus of freely moving rats. *Life Sci* 1992; 51(4): 285.

Maher, T. J., and Wurtman, R. J. Possible neurologic effects of aspartame, a widely used food additive. *Environ Health Perspect* 1987; 75: 53.

Manzoli, U., Rossi, E., Littarru, G. P., et al. Coenzyme Q_{10} in dilated cardiomyopathy. *Int J Tissue React* 1990; 12(3): 173.

Markstein, R. Hydergine: Interaction with the neurotransmitter systems in the central nervous system. *J Pharmacol* 1985; 3: 1.

Mathura, C. B., Singh, H. H., Tizabi, Y., Hughes, J. E., and Flesher, S. A. Effects of chronic tryptophan loading on serotonin (5-HT) levels in neonatal rat brain. *JAMA* 1986; 78(7): 645.

Maurer, I., Bernhard, A., and Zierz, S. Coenzyme Q_{10} and respiratory chain enzyme activities in hypertrophied human left ventricles with aortic valve stenosis. *Am J Cardiol* 1990; 66(4): 504.

Maurizi, C. P. The therapeutic potential for tryptophan and melatonin: Possible roles in depression, sleep, Alzheimer's disease and abnormal aging. *Med Hypotheses* 1990; 31(3): 233.

Meier, R. W. Effects of prolonged co-dergocrine mesylate (Hydergine) treatment on local cerebral glucose uptake in aged Fischer 344 rats. *Arch Gerontol Geriatr* 1986; 5(1): 65.

Melegh, B., Kerner, J., Sandor, A., Vinceller, M., and Kispal, G. Effects of oral L-carnitine supplementation in low-birth-weight premature infants maintained on human milk. *Biol Neonate* 1987; 51(4): 185.

Melegh B., Szucs, L., Kerner, J., and Sandor, A. Changes of plasma free amino acids and renal clearances in carnitines in premature infants during L-carnitine-supplemented human milk feeding. *J Pediatr Gastroenterol Nutr* 1988; 7(3): 424.

Meunier, S. M. C., Monnier, M., Colleaux, Y., Seve, B., and Henry, Y. Impact of dietary tryptophan and behavioral type on behavior, plasma cortisol, and brain metabolites of young pigs. *J Anim Sci* 1991; 69(9): 3689.

Milusheva, E. Sperlagh, B., Kiss, B., et al. Inhibitory effect of hypoxic condition on acetylcholine release is partly due to the effect of adenosine released from the tissue. *Brain Res Bull* 1990; 24(3): 369.

Minkler, P. E., Ingals, S. T., and Hoppel, C. L. Determination of total carnitine in human urine by high-performance liquid chromatography. *J Chromatogr* 1987; 420(2): 385.

Mistry, S. D., Tripathi, C. G., Bhavsar, V. H., and Kelkar, W. The effect of centrophenoxine at the skeletal neuromuscular junction. *Indian J Physiol Pharmacol* 1985; 29(2): 89.

Mitchell, J. B., and Stewart, J. Effects of castration, steroid replacement, and sexual experience on mesolimbic dopamine and sexual behaviors in the male rat. *Brain Res* 1989; 491(1): 116.

Mizuno, Y. [The role of oxygen free radicals in the aging of the brain]. *Nippon Ronen Igakkai Zasshi* 1990; 27(2): 182.

Moller, S. E. Tryptophan to competing amino acids ratio in depressive disorder: Relation to efficacy of antidepressive treatments. *Acta Psychiatr Scand Suppl* 1985: 325: 3.

Morales, A., Condra, M., Owen, J. A., et al. Is yohimbine effective in the treatment of organic impotence? Results of a controlled trial. *J Urol* (Baltimore) 1987; 137(6): 1168.

Moret, C., Pastrie, I., and Briley, M. Carnitine acetyltransferase activity is not changed with age in rat brain and human platelets. *Neurobiol Aging* 1990; 11(1): 57.

Mortensen, S. A., Vadhanavikit, S., Muratsu, K., and Folkers, K. Coenzyme Q_{10}: Clinical benefits with biochemical correlates suggesting a scientific breakthrough in the management of chronic heart failure. *Int J Tissue React* 1990; 12(3): 155.

Mosharrof, A. H., and Petkov, V. D. Effects of citicholine and of the combination citicholine + piracetam on the memory (experiments on mice). *Acta Physiol Pharmacol Bulg* 1990; 16(1): 25.

Murakami, E., Iwata, T., Hiwada, K., and Kokubu, T. Brain glutathione and blood pressure control. *J Cardiovasc Pharmacol* 1987; 12: S112.

Murakami, E., Hiwada, K., and Kokubu, T. The role of brain glutathione in blood pressure regulation. *Jpn Circ J* 1988; 52(11): 1299.

Nagai, K., and Suda, T. Realization of spontaneous healing function by carnosine. *Methods Find Exp Clin Pharmacol* 1988; 10(8): 497.

Nagasawa, H., Kogure, K., Kawashima, K., Ido, T., Itoh, M., and Hatazawa J. Effects of co-dergocrine mesylate (Hydergine) in multi-infarct dementia as evaluated by positron emission tomography. *Tohoku J Exp Med* 1990; 162(3): 225.

Nakano, C., Takashima, S., and Takeshita, K. Carnitine concentration during the development of human tissues. *Early Hum Dev* 1989; 19(1): 21.

Neri, B., Comparini, T., Miliani, A., et al. Protective effects of L-carnitine (Carnitene) on acute adriamycin and daunomycin cardiotoxicity in cancer patients: A preliminary report. *Clin Trials J* 1983; 20(2): 98.

Neumann, H. J., Hollnack, W., Hollnack, B., and Frommel, H. [Circadian rhythm studies on the prenatal toxic effect of cyclophosphamide and centrophenoxine in Wistar rats]. *Anat Anz* 1985; 160(5): 345.

Ng, L. T., and Anderson, G. H. Route of administration of tryptophan and tyrosine affects short-term food intake and plasma and brain amino acid concentrations in rats. *J Nutr* 1992; 122(2): 283.

Nicholson, C. D. Pharmacology of nootropics and metabolically active compounds in relation to their use in dementia. *Psychopharmacol* (Berlin) 1990; 101(2): 147.

Ogasahara, S., Engel, A. G., Frens, D., and Mack, D. Muscle coenzyme Q deficiency in familial mitochondrial encephalomyopathy. *Proc Natl Acad Sci U.S.A.* 1989; 86(7): 2379.

Ogita, K., and Yoneda, Y. Selective potentiation by L-cysteine of apparent binding activity of [3H]glutathione in synaptic membranes of rat brain. *Biochem Pharmacol* 1989; 38(9): 1499.

Olah, V. A., Balla, G., Balla, J., Szabolcs, A., and Karmazsin, L. An in vitro study of the hydroxyl scavenger effect of Cavinton. *Acta Paediatr Hung* 1990; 30(2): 309.

Oliveira, J. S., Muccilo, G., Scozzafave, N. F., and Maffia, L. G. Changes in myocardial norepinephrine levels in response to stress, exercise and aging in control and T. cruzi-infected rats. *Braz J Med Biol Res* 1986; 19(3): 367.

Olpe, H. R., Steinmann, M. W., and Jones, R. S. Comparative electrophysiological investigations with Hydergine and other psychogeriatric agents on corticol and subcortical structures. *J Pharmacol* 1985; 3: 65.

Olsen, I. Alterations of the mitochondrial respiratory chain in human dilated cardiomyopathy. *Eur Heart J* 1990; 11(6): 509.

Page, T. G., Ward, T. L., and Southern, L. L. Effect of chromium picolinate on growth and carcass characteristics of growing-finishing pigs. *J. Anim Sci* 1991; 69 (Supp 1).

Pap, Z., Ajtai, P. E., Drasoveanu, M., and Dunca, J. [Adjuvant treatment with the Hydergine-romergan cocktail in dyspneic severe acute pneumopathies]. *Rev Pediatr Obstet Gynecol Pediatr* 1987; 36(3): 285.

Parker, W. D. J., Oley, C. A., and Parks, J. K. Multiple defects of the respiratory chain including complex II in a family with myopathy and encephalopathy. *Biochem Biophys Res Commun* 1989; 163(2): 695.

Pasantes-Morales, H., Wright, C. E., and Guall, G. E. Protective effect of taurine, zinc, and tocopherol on retinol-induced damage in human lymphoblastoid cells. *J Nutr* 1987; 114: 2256.

Pavlik, A., and Pilar, J. Protection of cell proteins against free-radical attack by nootropic drugs: Scavenger effect of pyritinol confirmed by electron spin resonance spectroscopy. *Neuropharmacol* 1989; 28(6): 557.

Pek, G., Fulop, T., and Zs, N. I. Gerontopsychological studies using NAI

("Nurnberger Alters-Inventar") on patients with organic psychosyndrome (DSM III, Category 1) treated with centrophenoxine in a double blind, comparative, randomized clinical trial. *Arch Gerontol Geriatr* 1989; 9(1): 17.

Perry, T. L., Hansen, S., and Jones, K. Brain amino acids and glutathione in progressive supranuclear palsy. *Neurol* 1988; 38(6): 943.

Peters, R. I., and Lack, D. B. Audiogenic seizures and brain serotonin after L-tryptophan and p-chlorophenylalanine. *Exp Neurol* 1985; 90(3): 540.

Petkov, W., and Vuglenova, Y. Pharmacological restoration of scopolamine-impaired memory. *Acta Physiol Pharmacol Bulg* 1985; 11(3): 37.

Pfaus, J. G., and Phillips, A. G. Differential effects of dopamine receptor antagonists on the sexual behavior of male rats. *Psychopharmacol* (Berlin) 1989; 98(3): 363.

Pfaus, J. G., Damsma, G., Nomikos, G. G., et al. Sexual behavior enhances central dopamine transmission in the male rat. *Brain Res* 1990; 530(2): 345.

Pfaus, J. G., and Phillips, A. G. Role of dopamine in anticipatory and consummatory aspects of sexual behavior in the male rat. *Behav Neurosci* 1991; 105(5): 727.

Pinelli, A., Travulzio, S., Malvezzi, L., and Zecca, L. Potentiation of the analgesic effects of tryptophan by allopurinol in rats. *Arzneimittelforschung* 1991; 41(8): 809.

Plasky, P., Marcus, L., and Salzman, C. Effects of psychotropic drugs on memory: Part 2. *Hosp Community Psychiatry* 1988; 39(5): 501.

Pleim, E. T., Matochik, J. A., Barfield, R. J., and Auerbach, S. B. Correlation of dopamine release in the nucleus accumbens with masculine sexual behavior in rats. *Brain Res* 1990; 524(1): 160.

Pomerantz, S. M. Dopaminergic influences on male sexual behavior of rhesus monkeys: effects of dopamine agonists. *Pharmacol Biochem Behav* 1992; 41(3): 511.

Pope, H. G. J., Jonas, J. M., Hudson, J. I., and Kafka, M. P. Toxic reactions to the combination of monoamine oxidase inhibitors and tryptophan. *Am J Psychiatry* 1985; 142(4): 491.

Posner, J. D., and Landsberg, L. Lack of efficacy of Hydergine in Alzheimer's disease [letter, comment]. *N Engl J Med* 1991; 324(3): 197.

Pradalier, A., Launay, J. M., Soliman, M., et al. [Platelet release of dopamine in the common migraine attack (erratum appears in *Presse Med* 1987; 16(32): 1600)]. *Presse Med* 1987; 16(27): 1321.

Price, L. H., Ricaurte, G. A., Krystal, J. H., and Heninger, G. R. Neuroendocrine and mood responses to intravenous L-tryptophan in 3,4-methylenedioxymethamphetamine (MDMA) users. Preliminary observations. *Arch Gen Psychiatry* 1989; 46(1): 20.

Price, W. A., Zimmer, B., and Kucas, P. Serotonin syndrome: A case report. *J Clin Pharmacol* 1986; 26(1): 77.

Ravindranath, V., Shivakumar, B. R., and Anandatheerthavarada, H. K. Low glutathione levels in brain regions of aged rats. *Neurosci Lett* 1989; 101(2): 187.

Rebouche, C. J., Bosch, E. P., Chenard, C. A., Schabold, K. J., and Nelson, S. E. Utilization of dietary precursors for carnitine synthesis in human adults. *J Nutr* 1989; 119(12): 1907.

Reimherr, F. W., Byerley, W. F., Ward, M. F., Lebegue, B. J., and Wender, P. H. Sertraline, a selective inhibitor of serotonin uptake, for the treatment of outpatients with major depressive disorder. *Psychopharmacol Bull* 1988; 24(1): 200.

Ricci A., Amenta, D., Cavallotti, C., Rossodivita, I., and Amenta, F. Autoradiographic localization of peripheral [3H]-hydergine binding sites. *Arch Int Pharmacodyn Ther* 1990; 304: 75.

Rischke, R., and Kreiglstein, J. Protective effect of vinpocetine against brain damage caused by ischemia. *Jpn J Pharmacol* 1991; 56(3): 349.

Rivner, M. H., Shamsnia, M., Swift, T. R., et al. A defect in mitochondrial electron-transport activity (NADH-coenzyme Q oxidoreductase) in Leber's hereditary optic neuropathy. *N Engl J Med* 1989; 320(20): 1331.

Rodriguez, S. S., Alonso, dIP. C., Tutor, J. C., et al. Carnitine deficiency associated with anticonvulsant therapy. *Clin Chim Acta* 1989; 191(2): 175.

Rogemont, C., Sarda, N., Gharib, A., and Pacheco, H. Changes in the rat sleepwake cycle produced by D,L-beta-(1-naphthyl)alanine, a tryptophan analog. *Neurosci Lett* 1988; 93(2–3): 287.

Romero, R., Felip, A., Llibre, J. M., Bonet, J., and Caralps, A. Co-dergocrine mesylate (Hydergine) and hypertensive emergencies [letter]. *Nephron* 1989; 51(1): 127.

Rossaint, R., Falke, K. J., et al. Inhaled nitric oxide for the adult respiratory distress syndrome. *New Engl J Med* 1993; 328(6): 399.

Rouy, J. M., Douillon, A. M., Compan, B., and Wolmark, Y. Ergoloid mesylates ("Hydergine") in the treatment of mental deterioration in the elderly: A 6-month double-blind, placebo-controlled trial. *Curr Med Res Opin* 1989; 11(6): 380.

Roy, D., and Singh, R. Age-related change in the multiple unit activity of the rat brain parietal cortex and the effect of centrophenoxine. *Exp Gerontol* 1988; 23(3): 161.

Rybalchenko, V. K., Lukoshko, S. A., Ostrovskaia, G. V., and Kulikova, N. V. [The surface-active properties of dimethylethanolamine and its effect on the ecto-ATPase activity of plasma membranes]. *Bull Eksp Biol Med* 1991; 111(2): 157.

Sakagami, H., Kikuchi, K., Takeda, M., et al. Macrophage stimulation activity of antimicrobial N,N-dimethylaminoethyl paramylon. *In Vivo* 1991; 5(2): 101.

Sakai, M., Ashihara, M., Nishimura, T., and Nagatsu, I. Carnosine-like immunoreactivity in human olfactory mucosa. *Acta Otolaryngol* (Stockholm) 1990; 109(5–6): 450.

Saletu, B., Grunberger, J., and Anderer, R. On brain protection of co-dergocrine mesylate (Hydergine) against hypoxic hypoxidosis of different severity: Double-blind placebo-controlled quantitative EEG and psychometric studies. *Int J Clin Pharmacol Ther Toxicol* 1990; 28(12): 510.

Sato, Y., and Kumamoto, Y. [Psychological stress and sexual behavior in male rats. II. Effect of psychological stress on dopamine and its metabolites in the critical brain areas mediating sexual behavior]. *Nippon Hinyokika Gakkai Zasshi* 1992; 83(2): 212.

Schapira, A. H., Cooper, J. M., Dexter, D., Clark, J. B., Jenner, P., and Marsden, C. D. Mitochondrial complex I deficiency in Parkinson's disease. *J Neurochem* 1990; 54(3): 823.

Schapira, A. H., Cooper, J. M., Morgan, H. J. A., Landon, D. N., and Clark, J. B. Mitochondrial myopathy with a defect of mitochondrial-protein transport. *N Engl J Med* 1990; 323(1): 37.

Schapira, A. H., Holt, I. J., Sweeney, M., Harding, A. E., Jenner, P., and Marsden, C. D. Mitochondrial DNA analysis in Parkinson's disease. *Mov Disord* 1990; 5(4): 294.

Schinetti, M. L., and Mazzini, A. Effect of L-carnitine on human neutrophil activity. *Int J Tissue React* 1986; 8(3): 199.

Schmidt, J. Comparative studies on the anticonvulsant effectiveness of nootropic drugs in kindled rats. *Biomed Biochim Acta* 1990; 49(5): 413.

Schmidt, J. Influence of nootropic drugs on apomorphine-induced stereotyped behaviour in rats. *Biomed Biochim Acta* 1990; 49(1): 133.

Schneider, H. D. [Treatment of sleep disorders with L-tryptophan. Uses of interval therapy in severe insomnia and hypnotic dependence]. *Fortschr Med* 1987; 105(6): 113.

Schoenen, J., Gainko, J. S., and Lenaerts, M. Blood magnesium levels in migraine. *Ceohalalgia* 1991; 11: 87.

Schwartz, R. H., Gruenewald, P. J., Klitzner, M., and Fedio, P. Short-term memory impairment in cannabis-dependent adolescents. *Am J Dis Child* 1989; 143(10): 1214.

Semenova, T. P., Kozlovskaia, M. M., Gromova, E. A., and Valdman, A. V. [Characteristics of the action of psychostimulants on learning and memory in rats]. *Bull Eksp Biol Med* 1988; 106(8): 161.

Semsei, I., and Zs, N. I. Superoxide radical scavenging ability of centrophenoxine and its salt dependence in vitro. *J Free Radic Biol Med* 1985; 1(5–6): 403.

Sergio, W. Use of DMAE (2-dimethylaminoethanol) in the induction of lucid dreams. *Med Hypoth* 1988; 26(4): 255.

Serino, F., Citterio, F., Lippa, S., et al. Coenzyme Q, alpha tocopherol and delayed function in human kidney transplantation. *Transplant Proc* 1990; 22(4): 1375.

Shalev, D. P., Soffer, Y., and Lewin, L. M. Investigations on the motility of human spermatozoa in a defined medium in the presence of metabolic inhibitors and of carnitine. *Andrologia* 1986; 18(4): 368.

Sharonov, B. P., Govorova, N., and Lyzlova, S. N. Carnosine as a potential scavenger of oxidants generated by stimulated neutrophils. *Biochem Int* 1990; 21(1): 61.

Shiosaka, S. Attempts to make models for Alzheimer's disease. *Neurosci Res* 1992; 13(4): 237.

Shoaf, A. R., Jarmer, S., and Harbison, R. D. Heavy metal inhibition of carnitine acetyltransferase activity in human placental syncytiotrophoblast: Possible site of action of HgCl2, CH3HgCl, and CdCl2. *Teratogenesis Carcinog Mutagen* 1986; 6(5): 351.

Siegl, H. Renal and antihypertensive effects of co-dergocrine (Hydergine) in rats. *J Pharmacol* 1985; 3: 113.

Sigala, S., Imperato, A., Rizzonelli, P., Casolini, P., Missale, C., and Spano, P. L-alpha-glycerylphosphorylcholine antagonizes scopolamine-induced amnesia and enhances hippocampal cholinergic transmission in the rat. *Eur J Pharmacol* 1992; 211(3): 351.

Simic, M., and Jovanovic, S. V. Antioxidation mechanisms of uric acid. *J Am Chem Soc* 1989; 111: 5778.

Sindrup, S. H., Gram, L. F., Brosen, K. Eshoj, O., and Mogensen, E. F. The selective serotonin reuptake inhibitor paroxetine is effective in the treatment of diabetic neuropathy symptoms. *Pain* 1990; 42(2): 135.

Singh, R., Shepherd, I. M., Derrick, J. P., Ramsay, R. R., Sherratt, H. S., and Turnbull, D. M. A case of carnitine palmitoyltransferase II deficiency in human skeletal muscle. *Febs Lett* 1988; 241(1–2): 126.

Slivka, A., Mytilineou, C., and Cohen, G. Histochemical evaluation of glutathione in brain. *Brain Res* 1987; 409(2): 275.

Slivka, A., Spina, M. B., and Cohen, G. Reduced and oxidized glutathione in human and monkey brain. *Neurosci Lett* 1987; 74(1): 112.

Smiaek, M. Effect of reduced glutathione (GSH) on dopamine (DA) and gamma-aminobutyric acid (GABA) concentration in the mouse brain following intoxication with 1-methyl-4-phenyl-1,2,3,6-tetrahydropyridine (MPTP). *Neuropatol Pol* 1988; 26(3): 415.

Smidt, C. R., Steinberg, F. M., and Rucker, R. B. Physiologic importance of pyrroloquinoline quinone. *Proc Soc Exp Biol Med* 1991b 197(1), 19–26.

Smith, F. L., Yu, D. S., Smith, D. G., Leccese, A. P., and Lyness, W. H. Dietary tryptophan supplements attenuate amphetamine self-administration in the rat. *Pharmacol Biochem Behav* 1986; 25(4): 849.

Snyder, T. M., Little, B. W., Roman, C. G., and McQuillen, J. B. Successful treatment of familial idiopathic lipid storage myopathy with L-carnitine and modified lipid diet. *Neurol* 1982; 32(10): 1106.

Sofic, E., Riederer, P., Killian, W., and Rett, A. Reduced concentrations of ascorbic acid and glutathione in a single case of Rett syndrome: A postmortem brain study. *Brain Dev* 1987; 9(5): 529.

Sommi, R. W., Crismon, M. L., Bowden, C. L., et al. Fluoxetine: A serotonin-specific, second-generation antidepressant. *Pharmacother* 1987; 7(1): 1.

Spagnoli, L. G., Palmieri, G., Mauriello, A., et al. Morphometric evidence of the trophic effect of L-carnitine on human skeletal muscle. *Nephron* 1990; 55(1): 16.

Spinweber, C. L. L-tryptophan administered to chronic sleep-onset insomniacs: Late-appearing reduction of sleep latency. *Psychopharmacol* (Berlin) 1986; 90(2): 151.

Sprouse, J. S., Bradberry, C. W., Roth, R. H., and Aghajanian, G. K. 3,4-methylenedioxymethamphetamine-induced release of serotonin and inhibition of dorsal raphe cell firing: potentiation by L-tryptophan. *Eur J Pharmacol* 1990; 178(3): 313.

Squadrito, F., Sturniolo, R., Trimarchi, G. R., et al. Antihypertensive activity of indolepyruvic acid: A keto analogue of tryptophan. *J Cardiovasc Pharmacol* 1990; 15(1): 102.

Stancheva, S. L., and Alova, L. G. [Effect of centrophenoxine, piracetam and aniracetam on the monoamine oxidase activity in different brain structures of rats]. *Farmakol Toksikol* 1988; 51(3): 16.

Steers, W. D., McConnell, J., and Benson, G. S. Some pharmacologic effects of yohimbine on human and rabbit penis. *J Urol* (Baltimore) 1984; 131(4): 799.

Steurer, G., Fitscha, P., Ettl, K., and Sinzinger, H. Effects of Kydergine on platelet deposition on "active" human carotid artery lesions and platelet function. *Thromb Res* 1989; 55(5): 577.

Stith, I. E., Nag, S., Mukherjee, S., and Das, S. K. Effects of centrophenoxine on cholinephosphotransferase activity in maternal and fetal guinea pig lung. *Exp Lung Res* 1989; 15(4): 587.

Stocker, R. Yamamoto, Y., and McDonauch, A. F. Bilirubin is an antioxidant of possible physiological significance. *Science* 1987; 235: 1043.

Stoica, E., and Enulescu, O. Correction by centrophenoxine of abnormal catecholamine response to postural stimulus in patients with orthostatic hypotension due to brainstem ischemia. *Rom J Neurol Psychiatry* 1991; 29(3–4): 131.

Sun, I. L., Sun, E. E., Crane, F. L., and Moore, D. J. Evidence for coenzyme Q function in transplasma membrane electron transport. *Biochem Biophys Res Commun* 1990; 172(3): 979.

Sunamori, M., and Suzuki, A. Findings in muscle in complex I (NADH coenzyme Q reductase) deficiency. *Ann Neurol* 1988; 24(6): 749.

Takahashi, N., Iwasaka, T., Sugiura, T., et al. Effect of coenzyme Q_{10} on hemodynamic response to ocular timolol. *J Cardiovasc Pharmacol* 1989; 14(3): 462.

Tallal, P., Chase, C., Russell, G., and Schmitt, R. L. Evaluation of the efficacy of piracetam in treating information processing, reading and writing disorders in dyslexic children. *Int J Psychophysiol* 1986, 4(1): 41.

Tamura, T., Satoh, T., Minakami, H., and Tamada, T. Effect of Hydergine in hyperprolactinemia. *J Clin Endocrinol Metab* 1989; 69(2): 470.

Tareen, K. I., Bashir, A., Saeed, K., and Hussain, T. Clinical efficacy of co-dergocrine mesylate in children with learning difficulties. *J Int Med Res* 1988; 16(3): 204.

Tayarani, I., Cloez, I., Clement, M., Bourre, J. M. Antioxidant enzymes and related trace elements in aging brain capillaries and choroid plexus. *J Neuro-chem* 1989; 53(3): 817.

Terry, W. S., Phifer, B. Caffeine and memory performance on the AVLT. *J Clin Psychol* 1986; 42(6): 860.

Thienhaus, O. J., Wheeler, B. G., Simon, S. O., Zemlan, F. P., and Hartford, J. T. A controlled double-blind study of high-dose dihydroergotoxine mesylate (Hydergine) in mild dementia. *J Am Geriatr Soc* 1987; 35(3): 219.

Thompson, P., Huppert, F., and Trimble, M. Anticonvulsant drugs, cognitive function and memory. *Acta Neurol Scand* 1980; 80(75–81).

Thompson, T. L., Filley, C. M., Mitchell, W. D., Culig, K. M., LoVerde, M., and Byyny, R. L. Lack of efficacy of Hydergine in patients with Alzheimer's disease [published erratum appears in *N Engl J Med* 1990 Sept. 6; 323(10):691] [see comments]. *N Engl J Med* 1990; 323(7): 445.

Tibboel, D., Delemarre, F. M. C., Prazyrembel, H., Bos A. P., Affourtit, M. J., and Molenaar, J. C. Carnitine deficiency in surgical neonates receiving total paren-teral nutrition. *J Pediatr Surg* 1990; 25(4): 418.

Tipper, J., and Kaufman, S. Phenylalanine-induced phosphorylation and activa-tion of rat hepatic phenylalanine hydroxylase in vivo. *J Biol Chem* 1992; 267(2): 889.

Trevisan, C. P., Reichmann, H., DeVivo, D. C., and DiMauro, S. Beta-oxidation enzymes in normal human muscle and in muscle from a patient with an unusual form of myopathic carnitine deficiency. *Muscle Nerve* 1985; 8(8): 672.

Tristram, P. D., Eldershaw, T., Coluhoun, E. Q., Dora, K. A., et al. Pungent principles of ginger (Zingiber officinale) are thermogenic in the perfused rat hindlimb. *Int J Obesity* 1992; 16: 755.

Uysal, M., Jeyer-Uysal, M., Kocak-Toker, N., and Aykac, G. The effect of chronic ethanol ingestion on brain lipid peroxide and glutathione levels in rats. *Drug Alcohol Depend* 1986; 18(1): 73.

Uysal, M., Kutalp, G., Ozdemirler, G., and Aykac, G. Ethanol-induced changes in lipid peroxidation and glutathione content in rat brain. *Drug Alcohol Depend* 1989; 23(3): 227.

Volger, B. W. Alternatives in the treatment of memory loss in patients with Alzheimer's disease. *Clin Pharm* 1991; 10(6): 447.

Voronina, T. A., Garibova, T. L., Sopyev, Z., and Voronin, K. E. [Psychotropic properties of nootropic substances with a cholinergic action component in single and long-term use]. *Farmakol Toksikol* 1987; 50(5): 12.

Waber, L. J., Valle, D., Neill, C., et al. Carnitine deficiency presenting as familial cardiomyopathy: A treatable defect in carnitine transport. *J Pediatr* 1982; 101(5): 700.

Warner, R. K., Thompson, J. T., Markowski, V. P., et al. Microinjection of the dopamine antagonist cis-flupenthixol into the MPOA impairs copulation, penile reflexes and sexual motivation in male rats. *Brain Res* 1991; 540(1–2); 177.

Watanabe, H., Kobayashi, A., Hayashi, H., and Yamazaki, N. Effects of long-chain acyl carnitine on membrane fluidity of human erythrocytes. *Biochim Biophys Acta* 1989; 980(3): 315.

Weekley, L. B., Kimbrough, T. D., and Llewellyn, G. C. Disturbances in tryptophan metabolism in rats following chronic dietary aflatoxin treatment. *Drug Chem Toxicol* 1985; 8(3): 145.

Weissmann, D., Belin, M. F., Aguera, M., et al. Immunohistochemistry of tryptophan hydroxylase in the rat brain. *Neuroscience* 1987, 23(1): 291.

Willson, R. Free radical protection: Why vitamin E, not vitamin C, beta-carotene or glutathione? *Ciba Foundation Symposium 101* 1983; London (Pitman): 19.

Wilsher, C. R., Bennett, D., Chase, C. H., et al. Piracetam and dyslexia: Effects on reading tests. *J Clin Psychopharmacol* 1987; 7(4): 230.

Wood, W. G., Gorka, C., Armbrecht, H. J., Williamson, L. S., and Strong, R. Fluidizing effects of centrophenoxine in vitro on brain and liver membranes from different age groups of mice. *Life Sci* 1986, 39(22): 2089.

Worthley, L. I. G., Fishlock, R. C., and Snoswell, A. M. Carnitine deficiency with hyperbilirubinemia, generalized skeletal muscle weakness and reactive hypoglycemia in a patient on long-term total parenteral nutrition: Treatment with intravenous L-carnitine. *J Parenter Enter Nutr* 1983; 7(2): 176.

Wurtman, R. J. The choline-deficient diet [letter; comment]. *FASEB J,* 1991; 5(11), 2612.

Yamada, Y., Sugihara, K., Van, E. G. W., Roeijmans, H. J., and De, H. G. S. Human complex II (succinate-ubiquinone oxidoreductase): cDNA cloning of iron sulfur (lp) subunit of liver mitochondria. *Biochem Biophys Res Commun* 1990; 166(1): 101.

Yokogoshi, H., and Nomura, M. Effect of amino acid supplementation to a low-protein diet on brain neurotransmitters and memory-learning ability of rats. *Physiol Behav* 1991; 50(6): 1227.

Young, S. N. Acute effects of meals on brain tryptophan and serotonin in humans. *Adv Exp Med Biol* 1991; 294: 417.

Zhao, X. H., Kitamura, Y., and Nomura, Y. Age-related changes in NMDA-induced [3H]acetylcholine release from brain slices of senescence-accelerated mouse. *Int J Dev Neurosci* 1992; 10(2): 121.

Zierz, S., and Engel, A. G. Different sites of inhibition of carnitine palmitoyltransferase by malonyl-CoA, and by acetyl-CoA and CoA, in human skeletal muscle. *Biochem J* 1987; 245(1): 205.

Index